Acknowledgements

We would like to thank everybody who helped make this survey possible. First of all the other staff in Social Survey Division who contributed to the different stages of the survey including all the interviewers who carried out interviews with nurses and taught them how to complete the diary.

Secondly our thanks to the nursing officers in the 24 health districts who gave much enthusiastic support to the survey—providing lists of their staff and making arrangements for interviewing. The Family Practitioner Committees and Local Medical Committees also gave their support together with the general practitioners who provided the names of their employed nurses.

We are also grateful to colleagues in the Department of Health and Social Security who have provided support and assistance at all stages of the survey. Many professional associations and trade unions also gave their support.

Finally, of course, we must thank all the nurses who participated in the survey, for without their co-operation and hard work all our efforts would have been to no avail.

Contents

Index of tables

Four major variables are used throughout the report to analyse the data collected about nurses working in the community. The two basic variables are the type of nurse and the health district in which the nurse worked. The other two variables describe the way the nurses' work was organised—their attachment or patch working arrangements and the number of general practices they worked with. The index of tables has therefore been divided into three main sections—type of nurse, health district and work organisation—the major variable used in the table determines the section in which it is listed. Although the tables by attachment and number of practices worked with are not listed in the 'type of nurse' section they usually provide information for the four largest groups of nurses—district nurses, midwives, health visitors and auxiliaries.

Notes

On all tables percentages have been rounded so as to add up to 100%.

*denotes less than 0.5%.

— denotes no cases.

In general, in the text, attention has not been drawn to any difference which statistical tests suggest might have occurred by chance five or more times in 100.

Summary of findings

A systematic random sample of 25 health districts in England and Wales was selected. Twenty four of these agreed to participate. In these districts one in two of the district nurses and all the other nurses working in the community formed the national sample of 4528 nurses. Ninety-five per cent of these were interviewed; 85% were interviewed and also completed a diary of activities and patients seen for seven days. Fieldwork took place in March and April 1980 (Chapter 1).

One third of all nursing staff employed in the community were district nurses. Health visitors comprised one fifth. Midwives, including district nurse/midwives, the school nursing service and auxiliaries each made up one tenth of community nursing staff. Six per cent of the nurses were employed directly by general practitioners and three per cent were community psychiatric nurses. Geriatric, liaison and clinic nurses between them accounted for the last three per cent of staff (2.1).

More than 80% of district nurses, midwives, district nurse/midwives, health visitors, community psychiatric and liaison nurses worked full-time. At the other extreme only five per cent of family planning nurses were employed full-time (3.1).

District nurses, auxiliaries, midwives, district nurses/ midwives and health visitors could have a formal attachment to general practice. More than four fifths of them were attached. Full attachment, where nurses cared for all patients on particular GP lists only, was the most common form of attachment for each group of staff. Three other modified types of attachment were found where GP lists had been divided on a geographical basis and/or nurses worked an additional patch (3.2).

About one half of district nurses, district nurse/ midwives and health visitors worked with only one GP practice. But this applied to only 36% of auxiliaries and 20% of midwives. In contrast 34% of midwives and 19% of auxiliaries worked with four or more practices. This applied to 22% of district nurses and 14% of health visitors (3.2).

Nurses were asked to rate various aspects of their relationships with general practice, for example their opportunities to get to know GPs and discuss patients with doctors. These were found to vary by attachment and the number of practices worked with. Detailed analysis of data for district nurses, midwives and health visitors suggested that not being attached to general practice and working with a large number of practices were related to less positive assessments of relationships with general practice (5.5–5.8).

Nurses were also asked to rate six patient related aspects of their work, for example, opportunities to get to know clients/patients and continuity of patient care. These assessments were not related to patterns of attachment and patch working nor to the number of practices worked with (4.6).

Most nurses felt that the amount of travelling they did was 'about right'. However about one third of midwives, district nurse/midwives, community psychiatric and geriatric nurses felt that they did too much or far too much travelling. This was also true for one quarter of district nurses and health visitors. There was a slight tendency for attached nurses to view the amount of travel they did as excessive (6.1, 6.2). When information about actual travelling time from the diaries was compared there were no differences between attached and not attached district nurses, midwives and health visitors. However, small differences were observed for auxiliaries (6.5).

During the diary recording week more than one third of district nurses, midwives, district nurse/midwives, community psychiatric and geriatric nurses worked for 41 or more hours. This was also the case for more than one quarter of health visitors and liaison nurses. Most of these types of nurses worked full-time whereas more than half of family planning nurses worked on one day or less per week. Consequently three fifths of them had worked fewer than 11 hours during the week of diary recording (7.1, 7.2).

Only very small proportions of most types of nurses working in the community did any 'on call' duty. However, almost all midwives and district nurse/ midwives and one half of district nurses did 'on call' work. Of those who did some 'on call' work during diary recording midwives and district nurse/midwives were 'on call' for an average of 35 hours during the week. For district nurses the average was 21 hours (7.4).

From the diary recording nurses' working time can be divided into three main categories—travelling, non-clinical work and time with patients. District nurses spent 24% of their time travelling, 26% on non-clinical activities and 50% with patients. Midwives and district nurse/midwives had a similar pattern to district nurses but health visitors spent only 16% of their time travelling, 46% on non-clinical work and 38% with clients (Table 6.5).

The time spent with patients was divided into four broad categories—technical tests and assessments, for example, vision testing and ante-natal examinations; technical procedures, for example, injection and stitches; other nursing care, for example, bathing and personal care; and advisory activities. District nurses spent two fifths of their time with patients carrying out technical procedures, another two fifths on other nursing care and most of the remaining one fifth on advisory activities. Midwives, on the other hand, spent two fifths of their time with patients on technical tests and a third on advisory activities. Health visitors spent almost three quarters of their time with patients giving advice. Nursing auxiliaries spent 84% of their time with patients on other nursing care and only seven per cent on advisory activities. There was little variation between district nurses with different qualifications except that State Enrolled Nurses (SENs) without district training spent a higher proportion of their time on other nursing care than other district nurses (Table 9.2).

District nurses and auxiliaries spent about 90% of time with patients in patients' own homes. For midwives this proportion was less—66%—since 19% of their time was in clinics and 15% in other locations such as hospitals. Health visitors spent only 56% of their time with clients on home visits (8.2).

Overall women receive far more care than men from nurses working in the community. Midwives spent four fifths of their time with patients (excluding that in clinics), with women and the remaining one fifth with babies. Health visitors spent three fifths of their time with children—of the remainder nearly all was spent with women. District nurses spent two thirds of their time with women, auxiliaries three quarters. These last two groups of staff also spent three quarters of their time with patients aged 65 or more (8.4).

For most types of nurses the distribution of different kinds of non-clinical activities was similar. For example, health visitors spent 55% of their non-clinical time on clerical and administrative duties, 13% on telephone calls and 14% on meetings (10.1).

District nurses, midwives and district nurse/midwives did at least two fifths of their non-clinical work at home (10.3). These of course were the types of nurses who commonly worked from home rather than from a clinic or practice premises (3.3).

Fifty-seven per cent of health visitors had some assistance with their clerical work. Fewer, 15%, of district nurses and five per cent of midwives had such help (3.3). When all types of nurses were considered together nurses with clerical assistance spent a greater proportion of their time than nurses with no help on both non-clinical activities and on clerical and administrative work related to patients (10.4).

Amongst the 24 health districts which were included in the survey there were some striking differences. There was great variation between districts in the proportions of different types of nurses employed, although district nurses were always the largest group and health visitors the second largest. Only six districts had district nurse/midwives and two districts contained 62% of the geriatric nurses identified. Two districts had no family planning nurses and another two districts had no community psychiatric nurses (11.1).

From the diary information, rates were calculated for each health district to indicate the time spent with different age and sex groups per head of the population. The districts with the highest rates for time spent with the elderly were those districts which had a high proportion of staff who worked mainly with the elderly. These were also the districts with an above average proportion of elderly in the population (Table 11.5). Similarly districts with above average rates of time spent with schoolchildren were those which had high school nursing staffing ratios. More surprisingly, the districts which had high health visiting staff ratios were not the same districts as those with above average rates of time spent with young children (12.3).

Patterns of attachment and patch working also varied widely between the districts. In general the districts which had high attachment rates (over 80%) also had high proportions of nurses working 'full' attachment schemes whereas districts with low attachment rates had high proportions of nurses working only specific parts of a GP's list and/or working an additional geographical patch (11.2).

Districts with high attachment rates tended to have large proportions of nurses working with only one practice whereas districts with lower attachment rates were those where more nurses worked with large numbers of practices (11.3).

Nurses spent similar proportions of time on travelling in all the districts—nurses working in rural districts did not spend a greater proportion of their time on travelling (11.4). There was much more variation between districts in the proportion of time spent on non-clinical activity and amongst health visitors it seemed that those working in large cities spent most time on non-clinical activities (11.5).

The districts were grouped into six types according to a wide range of social and economic variables but in general the type of district seemed to have little bearing on most variables. The special characteristics and organisation of each particular district appeared to have a stronger effect (11.6).

1 Introduction

1.1 Reasons for the survey

A number of changes have taken place in the organisation and provision of community nursing in recent years and these changes have created a need for up to date, national information about community nurses and the work they are undertaking. This need is not met by the statistics collected routinely by the National Health Service. The Department of Health and Social Security therefore asked Social Survey Division of the Office of Population Censuses and Surveys to carry out a national survey of nurses working in the community.

Over the last few years there has been increased emphasis on providing health care in the community. Schemes such as those involving early discharge from hospital have an impact on the work carried out by district nurses. The trend away from home deliveries has affected the role of community midwives and has led to the development of schemes in some districts which enable commmunity midwives to work part-time in hospitals. Changes in legislation have brought school health and family planning services into the National Health Service, but little is known about them on a national basis. There has been a growth in the employment of specialist nurses, of State Enrolled Nurses (SENs) and of nursing auxiliaries which may alter the division of work between the various categories of nurses working in the community.

Over the last decade there has been a general movement towards the integration of community health services provided by doctors, nurses, other professionals and ancilliary staff. Multi-disciplinary primary health care teams have been established. Part of this movement has been the attachment of health authority nursing staff to general practitioners and a parallel increase in the direct employment of nurses by general practitioners.

On a wider front the altered demographic structure of the population and, in particular, the increase in the proportion of old people, is changing the need for community nursing services.

1.2 Aims of the survey

The purpose of the survey was three-fold. It first aimed to provide a profile of the nursing staff working in the community: their training, experience and qualifications, information on the way their work is organised and their attitudes towards it. Secondly it aimed to produce an outline of the activities carried out by the different types of nurses. This would include an analysis of the time spent on various categories of activity and relate this to the client groups being cared for. The third aim was to identify patterns of work within health districts and examine these patterns in relation to the characteristics of the health districts.

1.3 Coverage of the survey

Since the purpose of the survey was to describe the work carried out by nurses in the community it was important to cover all types of nurses and nursing auxiliaries. This meant that in addition to those nurses employed in the primary health care service, ie health visiting, district nursing and midwifery groups such as school health, family planning, clinic nurses, psychiatric, geriatric and other specialist nurses were included.

Most of the nurses working in the community are employed by health authorities, but in addition some GPs employ nurses directly to assist them in their practices. Practice nurses were included in the survey to provide a complete picture of community nursing in the selected districts. Other privately employed nurses were excluded.

The survey was of nurses who spent a proportion of their time on clinical duties. Thus nursing managers, that is, nursing officers and above, whose jobs were wholly administrative or supervisory were excluded, although nursing officers who were actually carrying out nursing duties in the community, for example, 'acting down' temporarily, were included in the survey. Clinic assistants who had no direct contact with patients but who carried out orderly-type duties were not included, nor were people employed by GPs on receptionist duties only, even if they had nursing qualifications.

Since the survey was of nurses working in the community, those working in hospitals and residential nurses in institutions such as schools and old people's homes were not eligible. However some nurses, especially midwives and particular groups of specialist nurses, combine working in hospitals with community work, and they were included.

1.4 Sample design

Since there is no national list of nurses working in the community it was necessary to select the sample in stages. Thus a sample of study areas was drawn and nurses working in these included in the survey. This had the advantage that the service in each area could be described and the work of different types of nurses could be related to characteristics of the study areas.

Health districts were chosen as the most appropriate study areas since they were the level within the health service at which community services are organised and therefore most nurses are likely to have clear identification with work in the district. Furthermore arrangements for interviewing could be conveniently carried out at this level.

The sample needed to be large enough to ensure that the main groups to be studied were of an adequate size to describe the work being done at a national level and also to allow comparisons between different kinds of districts.

It was decided to draw a sample of 25 health districts and within these districts to include all nurses working in the community. The exception was district nurses, a random half of whom were sampled since they formed by far the largest group.

Selection of health districts
A systematic random sample of health districts was drawn from a list of all health districts which were grouped in such a way as to ensure that the correct proportions of different kinds of districts were included and hence controlling the representativeness of the sample nationally. The following information was used for grouping (or 'stratifying') the districts:-

population size
the estimated age distribution of the population
region
metropolitan/non-metropolitan

Selection of nurses within districts
Having selected the sample of 25 health districts we contacted the district nursing officers in these districts to ask their permission to include health authority employed nurses in the survey and to make arrangements to obtain a list of the eligible nurses. One of the districts refused to participate in the survey so the report relates to nurses in the other 24 health districts.

The health districts provided us with a complete list of nurses eligible for inclusion, with the exception of practice nurses who are not employed by the health authorities.

It was estimated that the 24 co-operating health districts would yield approximately 5,700 eligible nursing staff. It was decided to take a random subsample of one half of the district nurses, which were the largest group of nurses in the community, since this reduced the cost of the survey but still provided adequate representation of district nurses.

The lists of nurses were compiled several weeks before interviewing began so it was necessary immediately the fieldwork started to check whether any staff changes had taken place. The survey was one of nurses in post in March 1980.

Selection of GP employed-practice nurses
Since practice nurses are employed by general practitioners and not the health authorities it was necessary to use a different approach. Firstly a list of the general practitioners working in the 24 selected health districts was obtained from the relevant Family Practitioner Committees. Then a letter explaining the method and purpose of the survey was sent to the (senior) general practitioner in each practice on the lists. The general practitioners were asked to complete a form giving the names of any nurses they employed directly. The letter explained that an interviewer would be contacting all the nurses to seek to interview them and to ask them to complete a diary of work activites for a week.

The response to this postal enquiry was high: 65% of the practices responded to the initial letter and a reminder brought the final response to 89%. The postal questionnaire identified 361 practice nurses.† Table 1.1 shows that 27% of practices employed one or more nurses.

Table 1.1 Number of practices employing nurses

Number of nurses employed	Percentage of practices
0	73
1	17
2	6
3	2
4	1
5 or more	1
Number of practices (= 100%)	*812*

It was noticeable that the doctors who replied quickly to our letter were more likely to employ nurses, this was probably because the survey seemed more relevant to them. At the pilot stage of the survey non-responding practices were telephoned. All of them reported having no employed nurses. It is not unreasonable to suppose, therefore, that the 11% who failed to respond contained a disproportionately high number of those doctors with no practice nurses.

1.5 Organisation of the survey
To meet the survey objectives information was collected from nurses in two different ways. Information about the nurses themselves was obtained by interview using Social Survey Division's trained interviewers. Information about the work they carried out was obtained by asking the nurses to complete a diary for seven days, recording their activities.

Interviewing began at the end of February 1980 and continued over the following two months. Each nurse was contacted individually by a Social Survey Division interviewer who arranged a time and place for interviewing that was convenient for that nurse. In some health districts the nursing officers had given instructions that the nurses were not to be contacted at home whilst in other districts it was administratively convenient and acceptable to the nursing staff to do this. The interview generally took between fifteen and twenty minutes, and covered questions on the nurse's job and its organisation,

---

†Some nurses were found at the interviewing stage to have vacated their post or not to be engaged in nursing duties.

2

qualifications, experience and training and nurses' views on some aspects of the work.

After the interview the interviewers explained how to use the diary by working through an example specific to each type of nurse, and leaving this example and the instructions with the nurse. Nurses were asked to complete the diary for each of seven days, irrespective of whether they were working on any or all of these days, beginning with the day following the interview.

Most research which has been done in the past on nurses working in the community has concentrated on just one type of nurse. The different research designs, questionnaires and diaries used make it difficult to contrast and compare the work of different types of nurses and to build a picture of the service as a whole. One strength of this survey is that the same documents were used for all kinds of staff in a nationally representative sample of health districts. The disadvantage of this was that the diary appeared fairly complicated since it had to cater for a wide range of duties. Although the diary took about half an hour on a working day to complete the time was very variable according to the type of job being carried out by the nurse. The interview and diary were extensively piloted amongst nurses in two health districts and were amended in the light of this experience.

Nurses were asked to fill in the diary during the day as they carried out their work but, of course, they may not all have done so. The pilot work had indicated, however, that most nurses kept fairly detailed time sheets which were useful in the diary compilation. Nurses were asked to return the diaries by post to the interviewers to save the cost of a further visit, but interviewers did call on nurses who failed to return a diary.

1.6 Research literature and survey document design
It is usual when reporting on research such as this to include a discussion of related published research findings at this stage and to refer to them for comparative purposes throughout the report. A very large number of reports, books and articles were read as a preparation for the survey. These covered the main research literature on the largest groups of nurses working in the community—district nurses and health visitors—as well as research that could be found on the smaller groups of staff such as GP employed nurses and school nurses. Since the main priority of the research was to produce the findings in a published form as quickly as possible we have made no attempt whatsoever in reporting the findings to relate them to the results of other enquiries. This anyway would have become laborious for both the writer and the reader since this survey covers all kinds of staff and the majority of previously published research covers only one type of nurse. Also our methodology—covering a national sample of all types of staff—makes difficult many comparisons with local studies or studies of one group of staff.

This introduction therefore does not include the usual literature review. However several studies were useful when designing the survey documents—particularly the important classifications of nursing activity and types of patients that were used on the diary. These classifications, which had to be used by all different kinds of nurses, were devised by taking the comparable classifications used in studies of particular types of staff, adding them together, removing and/or standardising any overlap, and balancing the fineness of detail so as not to collect more detailed information from one type of nurse than from another. This lengthy process was also aided by our advisers at the Department of Health and Social Security and in the Scottish Home and Health Department, by discussions with many contacts in both the nursing and research fields and by some of the professional associations whom we informed at the beginning of our work. Finally the classifications were tested and adapted as a result of the pilot survey.

The following reports were useful in the construction of classifications used for diary coding:

June Clark, 1973, *A family visitor. A descriptive analysis of health visiting in Berkshire,* Royal College of Nursing and National Council of Nurses of the United Kingdom.

Lizbeth Hockey, 1966, *Feeling the pulse,* Queen's Institute of District Nursing.

Lizbeth Hockey, 1968, *Care in the balance,* Queen's Institute of District Nursing.

Tyrell Marris, 1971, *The work of health visitors in London,* Greater London Research, Department of Planning and Transportation Report No. 12.

D Potter and Lizbeth Hockey, 1976, *District nurses in England,* Nursing Research Unit, University of Edinburgh.

Karin R Poulton, 1977, *Evaluation on community nursing service of Wandsworth and East Merton Teaching District,* Research Report, St George's Hospital, London SW17 0QT.

B L E C Reedy, A V Metcalfe, M de Roumanie, D J Newell, P R Philips, 1978, *Nurses and nursing in primary care in England, Phase 3—The characteristics and work of attached and employed nurses,* Medical Care Research Unit, University of Newcastle upon Tyne.

1.7 Response
Response of districts
As explained one of the 25 health districts originally selected for the survey refused to take part as its staff had recently co-operated in another study on community nursing which had involved the completion of diaries. It is estimated that about 160 nurses from this district would have been included in this survey.

Response of nurses
A sample of 4662 nurses was selected for interview including 361 practice nurses. Some nurses were found at the interviewing stage to be ineligible, usually because they were wholly employed on administrative or

receptionist duties or were resident nurses in institutions. The other category of ineligible staff consisted of nurses who had left their posts after the lists had been obtained from the districts but who had not been replaced at the time of interviewing. Thus 4528 nurses were identified as eligible for inclusion in the survey.

Table 1.2 gives these figures and the reasons for non-response. Only two per cent of nurses refused to participate in the survey and a further three per cent could not be contacted or interviewed within the field period. Thus the proportion of eligible nurses who were interviewed was 95%. However 10% of those who were interviewed either refused to complete the diary or never returned it to the interviewer. This gives a response rate to both the interview and diary of 85%. Thirty-five diaries had to be rejected as they were incompleted or unseable for other reasons.

Table 1.2 Response of nurses to the interview and diary

	Number	%
Nurses selected after sub-sampling district nurses	4662	
Ineligible—not community nurses	46	
—nurses who had left	87	
Eligible for interview	4528	100
Non-response—non-contacts	151	3
—refusals	74	2
Interview and diary completed	3861 } 4303	85 } 95
Interview only completed	442	10

Variation between health districts
Table 1.3 shows the response for each of the 24 health districts. Response to the interview, as shown by the bracketed figures varied from 89% to 99% with ten of the districts achieving a response rate of 97% or above. Response rates to both interview and diary varied more

widely—from 70% to 96%. However 21 of the districts achieved response to both parts of the survey of 80% or more. The very high response rates occurred in districts where support at management level was very strong and nurses were given a great deal of encouragement to take part. Lower response rates were commonly caused by groups of nurses who worked together deciding to refuse to participate or being difficult to contact.

Variation between different types of nurses
The response of the different types of nurses identified in the survey are shown at Table 1.4. Response to the interview varied from 91% of clinic nurses to 100% of liaison nurses—both very small groups. Among the large groups of staff response was very similar—94% of district nurses were interviewed, 96% of health visitors and 97% of auxiliaries. As with health districts the response to both interview and diary varied more widely from 79% among midwives to 96% among liaison nurses.

1.8 Plan of the report
Having discussed the background to and the methodology of the survey the report now goes on to describe the findings. Chapters 2 to 5 concentrate on information collected during the interviews with nurses, the first two covering basic factual details such as personal characteristics, qualifications and work organisation. Chapter 4 describes nurses answers to a series of attitude questions related to client/patient aspects of their work while Chapter 5 looks in greater detail at relationships with other primary health care staff—general practice in particular.

The next two chapters combine questionnaire and diary information and consider travelling and hours worked. Chapters 8 to 10 deal exclusively with diary data and describe the activities carried out by nurses and the time spent with different kinds of clients/patients.

Table 1.3 Response rates for the 24 health districts

	1	2	3	4	5	6	7	8	9	10	11	12	13	14	15	16	17	18	19	20	21	22	23	24	All
	%	%	%	%	%	%	%	%	%	%	%	%	%	%	%	%	%	%	%	%	%	%	%	%	%
Non-response																									
– non-contact	4	7	2	9	3	1	8	2	2	5	1	8	1	4	2	6	3	—	6	1	3	1	2	3	3
– refusal	4	—	—	2	3	2	1	3	1	3	—	1	2	1	1	1	1	1	2	1	1	2	—	2	2
Interview and diary completed	80 } 92	89 } 93	86 } 98	70 } 89	83 } 94	86 } 97	74 } 91	85 } 95	90 } 97	71 } 92	94 } 99	82 } 91	83 } 97	84 } 95	89 } 97	88 } 93	89 } 96	96 } 99	86 } 92	90 } 98	88 } 96	91 } 97	90 } 98	86 } 95	85 } 95
Interview only completed	12	4	12	19	11	11	17	10	7	21	5	9	14	11	8	5	7	3	6	8	8	6	8	9	10
Proportion of those interviewed who completed diary	87%	96%	88%	79%	88%	89%	81%	89%	93%	77%	95%	90%	86%	88%	92%	95%	93%	97%	93%	92%	92%	94%	92%	91%	90%
Eligible for interview (= 100%)	*171*	*193*	*171*	*114*	*219*	*186*	*191*	*154*	*291*	*168*	*178*	*196*	*141*	*233*	*230*	*97*	*155*	*108*	*173*	*118*	*302*	*237*	*185*	*317*	*4528*

Table 1.4 Response rates for different types of nurses

	All DN	Auxil-iaries	GP empl.	Mid-wives	DN/Midw.	HV†	Schl.† Nurse	Fam. Plan	Comm. Psych.	Geria-tric	Liai-son	Clinic	All Nurses
	%	%	%	%	%	%	%	%	%	%	%	%	%
Non-response – non-contact	4	2	8	5	3	2	2	4	2	—	—	5	3
– refusal	2	1	*	1	4	2	—	4	2	8	—	4	2
Interview and diary completed	84 } 94	86 } 97	80 } 92	79 } 94	83 } 93	88 } 96	90 } 98	86 } 92	83 } 96	82 } 92	96 } 100	84 } 91	85 } 95
Interview only completed	10	11	12	15	10	8	8	6	13	10	4	7	10
Proportion of those interviewed who completed diary	90%	89%	87%	84%	89%	92%	92%	94%	86%	89%	96%	92%	90%
Eligible for interview (= 100%)	*880*	*631*	*316*	*395*	*109*	*1170*	*494*	*236*	*142*	*48*	*50*	*57*	*4528*

†*Health visitors and school nurse assistants have been considered with health visitors and school nurses in this table because interviewers did not record assistants separately on the non-response sheets.*

The final two chapters explore similarities and differences between the 24 health districts and look at relationships between staffing ratios and actual amounts of time spent with clients/patients.

The very first task of the findings is to describe the kinds of nurses who worked in the community. In all we identified fourteen different kinds of nurses. Where appropriate information for each of these is given in all the tables of the report. However it is impossible to mention each type of nurse in relation to every subsection of the text. Readers interested in one particular type of nurse can of course collate all the relevant findings from the tables.

2 Characteristics of nurses working in the community

This first chapter of results begins by showing the different types of nurses employed in the community in the sample of health districts included in the survey. It then looks at some basic characteristics of the different types of nurses such as their age, sex and marital status; their qualifications training and experience.

2.1 Types of nurses

Table 2.1 shows how this national sample of nurses working in the community was distributed between the different types of staff. Column a of the table shows the distribution for all staff employed in the districts at the time of the survey and therefore includes the five per cent who either refused to take part or who could not be contacted. Column b shows figures for those staff who were interviewed. As can be seen there was little difference between the two distributions. In the table the number of district nurses interviewed have been doubled so that they are correctly represented. Only one in two of the district nurses were selected for interview.

The first question nurses were asked in the interview was 'Which of the categories of community work best describes your main job?' They were handed a card containing 15 categories.† There were so few staff who described themselves as bath attendants and night sitters that they have been included with nursing auxiliaries. Two extra categories of staff that could not be otherwise included identified themselves at this question— one was joint duty district nurse/midwives and the other was clinic nurses.

Although we expected to find joint duty district nurse/health visitors, particularly in rural areas, none identified themselves in the districts in the survey.

District nurses and district nurse assistants were divided into four categories depending on their qualifications ie SRN plus a district nursing qualification, SRNs without, SENs with a district nursing qualification and SENs without. There were seven assistants who had no basic nursing qualifications. These were added to the auxiliary group. (Only 26 nurses identified themselves as district nurse assistants.)

Table 2.1 shows that one third of all staff employed in the community were district nurses. More than one half of these were district trained SRNs, the remainder either untrained (for the district) SRNs or SENs. Just over one tenth of all staff were nursing auxiliairies. Midwives and

---

†See Q1 at questionnaire in Appendix I.

Table 2.1 Types of nurses employed in the community—based on number of staff in post and number of staff who were interviewed

Type of nurse†	a Staff in post	b Staff interviewed
	%	%
DN SRN+	17	18
DN SRN–	6	7
DN SEN+	5 } 33	5 } 32
DN SEN–	3	2
DN NR	2	–
Midwives	8	7
District nurse/midwives	2	2
Health visitors	20	20
Health visitor assistants	1	1
Auxiliaries, etc	11	12
GP employed nurses	6	6
School nurses	8	9
School nurse assistants	1	1
Family planning	4	4
Community psychiatric	3	3
Geriatric nurses	1	1
Liaison nurses	1	1
Clinic nurses	1	1
Number of nurses (=100%)	*5401*	*5132*

†DN SRN+   *District nurse SRN with district training*
DN SRN–   *District nurse SRN without district training*
DN SEN+   *District nurse SEN with district training*
DN SEN–   *District nurse SEN without district training*
DN NR   *Column a of the table includes the 5% of nurses who did not respond to the survey—we knew which type of nurses they were except that we did not know the qualifications of the district nurses.*

NB *The number of district nurses interviewed has been doubled in this table since only one in two of them were selected for interview.*

district nurse/midwives accounted for another tenth of the staff, the school nursing service a further tenth. Health visitors and their assistants comprised the second largest group— one fifth of all staff. Six per cent of the nurses were employed directly by general practitioners and three per cent were community psychiatric nurses. Geriatric, liaison and clinic nurses between them accounted for the last three per cent of staff.

Further details on full-time equivalents and variations betwen the districts are discussed in Chapter 11.

2.2 Sex, age and marital status

Nurses working in the community are predominantly female and there were no male midwives, district nurse/midwives or family planning nurses in our sample. Table 2.2 shows that there was a very small proportion of men amongst most types of nurses except for community psychiatric nurses and liaison nurses—60% of community psychiatric nurses were male and 14% of liaison nurses. Four per cent of the district nurses were male. A total of 148 male nurses were interviewed.

Table 2.3 shows the age distributions of the different types of nurses. The basic pattern of these distributions is for about one third of nurses to fall into the 30-39 age-group, another third into the 40-49 group and the remaining third to be evenly spread between the 20-29 and 50-59 groups. The exceptions to this basic pattern were community psychiatric nurses who were younger than the norm and school nurses, family planning nurses, geriatric nurses and auxiliaries who tended to be older. District nurses without district training were younger than their colleagues with post basic training.

The types of nurses with smaller than average proportions in the younger age groups also tended to have larger proportions who were married. This can be seen from Table 2.4. The majority of nurses were married although one quarter of midwives and health visitors were single.

2.3 Qualifications and training

Table 2.5 shows the proportion of nurses with various nursing qualifications. All nurses except auxiliaries were asked about their qualifications.† The qualifications held varied considerably for the different types of nurses. Looking first at basic qualifications, all health visitors and very high proportions of family planning nurses and district nurse/midwives were SRNs. Most GP employed practice nurses, school nurses, health visitor assistants, geriatric nurses and liaison nurses were either SRN or SEN. The RMN qualification was held by 88% of community psychiatric nurses. Ten per cent of liaison nurses also had RMN. Eighty-three per cent of school nurse assistants and 14% of clinic nurses had no qualifications.

† Q22 Nurses were asked 'What nursing qualifications do you have?' and handed a card listing the qualifications set out in the questionnaire.

Table 2.2 Type of nurse by sex

Sex of nurse	All DNs	DN SRN+	DN SRN −	DN SEN+	DN SEN −	Auxil-iaries	GP empl.	Mid-wives	DN/Midw.	HV	HV ass.	Schl. Nurse	Sch.N ass.	Fam. Plan.	Comm. Psych.	Geri-atric	Liai-son	Clinic
	%	%	%	%	%	%	%	%	%	%	%	%	%	%	%	%	%	%
Female	96	95	96	97	95	99	99	100	100	99	99	100	100	100	40	98	86	96
Male	4	5	4	3	5	1	1	—	—	1	1	—	—	—	60	2	14	4
Number of nurses (= 100%)	824	457	171	132	64	609	291	371	102	1057	67	442	42	221	136	44	50	52

Table 2.3 Type of nurse by age

Age-group	All DNs	DN SRN+	DN SRN −	DN SEN+	DN SEN −	Auxil-iaries	GP empl.	Mid-wives	DN/Midw.	HV	HV ass.	Schl. Nurse	Sch.N ass.	Fam. Plan.	Comm. Psych.	Geri-atric	Liai-son	Clinic
	%	%	%	%	%	%	%	%	%	%	%	%	%	%	%	%	%	%
Under 20 years	—	—	—	—	1	1	—	—	—	—	—	—	—	—	—	—	—	6
20 – 29 years	15	10	20	13	33	3	11	11	16	12	5	5	10	5	23	2	14	10
30 – 39 years	33	31	44	25	36	35	25	35	28	26	28	31	29	34	43	31	26	33
40 – 49 years	34	37	28	38	16	37	34	34	42	36	37	46	45	36	24	37	36	23
50 – 59 years	17	21	8	22	13	21	25	19	13	24	27	17	14	23	10	28	20	27
60 or more years	1	1	*	2	1	3	5	1	1	1	3	1	2	2	1	2	4	2
Number of nurses (= 100%)	824	457	171	132	64	609	291	371	102	1057	67	442	42	221	136	44	50	52

Table 2.4 Type of nurse by marital status

Marital status	All DNs	DN SRN+	DN SRN −	DN SEN+	DN SEN −	Auxil-iaries	GP empl.	Mid-wives	DN/Midw.	HV	HV ass.	Schl. Nurse	Sch.N ass.	Fam. Plan.	Comm. Psych.	Geri-atric	Liai-son	Clinic
	%	%	%	%	%	%	%	%	%	%	%	%	%	%	%	%	%	%
Married	76	78	83	67	71	85	85	65	73	66	75	85	82	96	74	80	66	75
Single	13	12	11	16	17	3	7	25	20	24	12	6	7	*	18	14	24	13
Widowed	3	3	1	4	3	6	3	3	1	3	8	4	7	2	1	2	6	2
Divorced	6	6	5	8	6	6	3	5	3	5	1	4	2	2	4	4	2	8
Separated	2	1	—	5	3	*	2	2	3	2	4	1	2	*	3	—	2	2
Number of nurses (= 100%)	824	457	171	132	64	609	291	371	102	1057	67	442	42	221	136	44	50	52

Table 2.5 Type of nurse by nursing qualifications

Nursing qualifications	All DNs	DN SRN+	DN SRN −	DN SEN+	DN SEN −	GP empl.	Mid-wives	DN/Midw.	HV	HV ass	Schl. Nurse	Sch.N ass.	Fam. Plan.	Comm. Psych.	Geri-atric	Liai-son	Clinic
	%	%	%	%	%	%	%	%	%	%	%	%	%	%	%	%	%
SRN or RGN	76	100	100	—*	—	87	73	96	100	80	88	—	98	38	86	86	80
SEN	27	4	4	100	100	13	12	5	4	25	8	10	5	10	9	10	6
RMN	2	3	2	1	1	1	*	2	2	3	1	2	*	88	2	10	4
SCM or CMB Pt 1	25	32	36	1	—	28	99	99	70	29	27	—	38	2	30	30	20
RSCN or RFN	5	5	9	—	3	6	4	6	6	8	12	—	5	1	7	10	4
HV certificate	1	1	3	—	—	2	*	4	99	3	3	—	10	—	2	8	—
District nursing certificates	61	83	—	95	—	5	6	47	8	8	3	—	3	2	26	48	6
QIDN	12	20	—	6	—	4	7	29	9	5	3	—	1	—	5	14	—
BTA certificate	3	3	3	2	2	1	2	3	1	1	1	—	1	—	5	8	4
Obstetrics certificate	6	6	9	1	3	3	2	5	23	6	5	—	8	1	5	6	10
Orthopaedics certificate	2	2	4	1	1	3	3	1	3	2	15	—	96	—	12	4	10
Family planning certificate	4	6	4	1	—	13	26	10	18	6	15	—	96	—	12	4	10
Health education certificate	*	1	—	—	—	—	1	1	4	—	1	—	1	—	—	—	—
Nursery nurse/NNEB	*	*	1	—	—	1	4	1	1	3	2	—	2	—	2	2	4
Community psychiatry	—	—	—	—	—	—	—	—	—	—	—	—	—	15	—	—	—
Diploma in nursing	1	2	1	—	—	1	1	2	1	—	*	—	1	—	1	4	—
Other diplomas	5	6	8	2	2	6	6	5	7	8	8	2	4	8	5	12	10
Other qualifications	1	*	1	2	3	*	1	3	2	1	1	5	1	16	5	2	—
None	—	—	—	—	—	—	—	—	—	—	—	83	—	—	2	—	14
Number of nurses (= 100%)	824	457	171	132	64	291	371	102	1057	67	442	42	221	136	44	50	52

Amongst the post registration qualifications the family planning certificate, the midwifery qualifications (SCM or CMB Pt 1) and the district nursing certificates (including QIDN) were the most common even where they were not directly related to the nurse's current job.

Sixty-one per cent of all district nurses had one of the district nursing certificates and 12% had the QIDN, with 25% also holding a midwifery qualification. A smaller proportion of the midwives had the basic SRN/SEN qualifications but 99%* had the SCM or CMB Pt 1 and two per cent had an obstetrics certificate. One quarter of the midwives also held a family planning qualification. Joint duty district nurse/midwives held similar qualifications to the midwives but in addition three quarters had a district nursing qualification.

Nearly all (99%)† health visitors had a health visitors certificate. A very high proportion also had a midwifery or obstetrics qualification and nearly a fifth had a family planning certificate.

GP employed practice nurses, school nurses, geriatric, liaison and clinic nurses all had a similar pattern of qualifications with high proportions being SRN or SEN and between 20% and 30% also having a midwifery qualification. Small proportions of these nurses held other kinds of qualifications. However 31% of geriatric nurses and 62% of liaison nurses had a district nursing training. Only 9% of GP employed practice nurses had a district nursing qualification.

---

* Midwives cannot practice without a recognised midwifery qualification. The questionnaires of the one per cent who did not have one were examined. All but one of these nurses were recorded as having an obstetrics certificate. The other was, from other questions, definitely working as a midwife. It is possible that either the nurse or the interviewer made an error in the interview.

†The questionnaires of the one per cent who did not have a health visitors certificate were examined. On about half of them it appeared that either the nurse or the interviewer had made an error; the other half were rather unusual types of health visitor and would perhaps not be strictly defined as health visitors.

Nurses were asked 'Do you have a teaching instructors or tutors certificate or any other job related qualifications?' Table 2.6 shows that the different types of nurses held different types of teaching certificates. For example, 22% of district trained SRN district nurses held a practical work teachers certificate, 16% of midwives a midwifery teaching certificate, 20% of health visitors a field work certificate and 42% of family planning nurses were qualified as instructing nurses.

Table 2.7 shows the proportions of nurses who had been on management courses since starting their current job. Among district nurses only small proportions of SRNs without district training and SENs had been on management courses. This was also true for health visitor assistants, GP nurses, school, family planning and clinic nurses. Between one third and one half of the other types of nurses had some management training in their current job.

All staff, were asked about refresher courses and in-service training during their current job. Nurses employed by GPs were much less likely than Area Health Authority staff to have had this kind of training. Only one quarter of them reported some compared with an average of three quarters of the other staff. The detailed answers to the question are shown in Table 2.8. Refresher courses, on the job training and study days on specific conditions were the most commonly mentioned by all groups of nurses.

2.4 Experience in the community
Table 2.9 shows the length of time that nurses had worked (as that particular type of nurse) in the community. Looking first at district nurses one half had been in the community for five years or more. However nurses with district training had much longer experience in the community that those without, about a third of the latter had worked as a district nurse for less than one year.

District nurse SRNs with district training were very similar to midwives and health visitors in having long

Table 2.6 Teaching instructions, tutors certificate or other job related qualifications, by type of nurse

Type of qualification	All DNs	DN SRN+	DN SRN −	DN SEN+	DN SEN −	GP empl.	Mid-wives	DN/Midw.	HV	Schl. Nurse	Fam. Plan.	Comm. Psych.	Geri-atric	Liai-son	Clinic
	%	%	%	%	%	%	%	%	%	%	%	%	%	%	%
Health visitor tutor	—	—	—	—	—	—	—	—	—	*	—	—	—	—	—
District nurse tutor	—	—	—	—	—	—	1	1	—	—	—	—	—	—	—
Midwifery teachers certificate	*	*	—	—	—	*	16	2	*	*	*	—	—	—	—
Practical work teachers certificate	13	22	2	—	—	2	6	8	1	*	1	4	5	21	4
Field work certificate	*	*	1	—	—	—	1	—	20	—	1	2	—	—	—
Instructing nurse	*	*	—	—	—	1	3	—	1	2	42	1	2	—	2
Community Health nurse certificate	1	1	—	2	2	—	1	—	*	—	—	—	—	—	—
City and Guilds further education teaching certificate	*	*	1	—	—	—	*	—	3	*	1	1	—	6	—
Other	1	1	1	—	—	2	2	1	2	3	4	2	—	—	—
Proportion with qualification	15	24	4	2	2	5	28	12	25	4	45	12	9	27	6
Number of nurses (= 100%)	824	457	171	132	64	291	371	102	1057	442	221	136	44	50	52

Table 2.7 Attendance at management courses in current job, by type of nurse

	All DNs	DN SRN+	DN SRN −	DN SEN+	DN SEN −	GP empl.	Mid-wives	DN/Midw.	HV	HV ass.	Schl. Nurse	Fam. Plan.	Comm. Psych.	Geri-atric	Liai-son	Clinic
	%	%	%	%	%	%	%	%	%	%	%	%	%	%	%	%
Proportion who had attended management courses in current job	30	47	8	13	4	4	46	41	43	6	9	7	33	30	34	—
Number of nurses (= 100%)	824	457	17	132	64	291	371	103	1057	67	442	221	136	44	50	52

community experience. About one fifth had been in the community for fifteen years or more.

Family planning nurses as a group had the highest proportion who had worked for five years or more, 69%. In contrast community psychiatric and liaison nurses had the shortest experience—nor surprising since many of their posts have only been created in recent years.

GP nurses, school, geriatric, clinic nurses and auxiliaries fell midway between the extremes with between 31% and 45% having five or more years experience.

Nurses were asked whether they had any experience in the community in nursing jobs that were different from their current one. Table 2.10 shows the proportions who had previously worked in the main areas of community nursing. Most of the nurses had no experience of this kind. Of the experience reported, district nursing and midwifery were most common.

Twenty-three per cent of health visitors had previous experience as district nurses, 28% as midwives and 15% as school nurses. Of GP employed nurses 18% had been district nurses, 9% midwives and 2% health visitors. A high proportion, 64% of liaison nurses had previously been district nurses. This was true for a substantial but much smaller proportion, 27%, of geriatric nurses.

Table 2.8 Attendance at refresher course or in service training in current job, by type of nurse

Type of course	All DNs	DN SRN+	DN SRN −	DN SEN+	DN SEN −	Auxil- iaries	GP empl.	Mid- Wives	DN/ Midw.	HV	HV ass.	Schl. Nurse	Sch.N ass.	Fam. Plan.	Comm. Psych.	Geri- atric	Liai- son	Clinic
	%	%	%	%	%	%	%	%	%	%	%	%	%	%	%	%	%	%
Refresher courses	31	40	18	22	16	23	8	78	64	42	16	25	10	48	9	26	16	9
Health education	4	6	2	2	2	2	—	6	4	17	6	18	2	4	1	7	2	4
Parentcraft	2	2	*	—	1	—	*	37	15	10	2	1	—	1	—	—	—	—
Audiometry and audio visual screening	1	1	1	1	—	1	*	—	1	28	13	24	14	—	—	5	4	6
Study days on specific conditions	36	45	19	35	25	23	8	12	30	29	31	35	17	22	27	37	46	11
Red Cross proficiency cert.	1	1	1	3	—	4	1	1	—	—	—	1	2	—	—	—	—	6
General or community nursing	12	12	12	13	9	13	*	—	7	*	4	2	12	—	8	12	10	4
On the job training	12	11	15	11	18	24	5	5	8	7	27	20	29	11	14	16	14	15
School nursing	*	—	—	1	—	—	—	—	—	*	4	10	2	—	—	2	—	—
Family planning	1	1	—	—	—	—	3	3	—	2	—	1	—	7	—	—	—	2
Counselling	*	—	—	2	—	—	—	*	—	1	3	1	—	1	1	—	—	—
Non-accidental injury	*	*	—	1	—	—	—	*	—	*	—	—	—	—	—	—	—	—
Relationships	—	—	—	—	—	—	—	—	—	*	—	—	—	—	—	1	—	—
Non-nursing	*	*	—	—	—	*	1	*	—	1	—	*	—	—	2	—	—	—
Other	5	6	6	1	5	5	4	3	4	2	2	3	2	2	9	5	8	6
Proportion who have done such training	71	81	53	68	53	71	26	87	87	83	75	87	64	71	54	77	80	46
Number of nurses (= 100%)	824	457	171	132	64	609	291	371	102	1057	67	442	42	221	136	44	50	52

Table 2.9 Length of time nurses had worked in the community as the type of nurse they currently were†

Number of years	All DNs	DN SRN+	DN SRN −	DN SEN+	DN SEN −	Auxil- iaries	GP empl.	Mid- wives	DN/ Midw.	HV	HV ass.	Schl. Nurse	Sch.N ass.	Fam. Plan.	Comm. Psych.	Geri- atric	Liai- son	Clinic
	%	%	%	%	%	%	%	%	%	%	%	%	%	%	%	%	%	%
Less than 1 year	12	2	38	1	31	16	19	10	11	10	25	14	17	6	31	23	26	29
1 year but less than 5 years	37	32	42	46	49	44	39	30	38	32	43	40	45	25	50	34	50	39
5 years but less than 10 years	28	33	14	38	14	30	22	26	14	25	18	30	31	34	18	30	24	14
10 years but less than 15 years	12	16	5	11	4	8	14	13	14	13	12	10	3	22	1	7	—	12
15 years but less than 20 years	7	10	*	3	1	2	3	11	9	11	—	5	2	10	—	6	—	4
20 years or more	4	7	1	1	1	*	3	10	14	9	2	1	2	3	—	—	—	2
Number of nurses (= 100%)	824	457	171	132	64	609	291	371	102	1057	67	442	42	221	136	44	50	52

†*Q2: How many years altogether have you worked as a [type of nurse] in the community?*

Table 2.10 Previous experience in other community nursing jobs, by type of nurse

Experience in the community at any level	All DNs	DN SRN+	DN SRN −	DN SEN+	DN SEN −	Auxil- iaries	GP empl.	Mid- wives	DN/ midw.	HV	HV ass.	Schl. Nurse	Sch.N ass.	Fam. Plan.	Comm. Psych.	Geri- atric	Liai- son	Clinic
	%	%	%	%	%	%	%	%	%	%	%	%	%	%	%	%	%	%
None	72	70	61	86	86	89	63	73	71	37	59	64	76	53	74	55	22	62
District nurse	/	/	/	/	/	1	18	18	6	23	20	13	—	10	4	27	64	17
Midwife	10	14	13	—	—	—	9	/	12	28	3	7	—	12	2	11	10	6
Health visitor	1	1	3	—	—	*	2	*	3	/	3	2	—	9	—	2	6	—
Health visitor assistant	1	1	1	—	—	*	1	1	1	5	/	4	2	3	—	—	8	2
School nurse	5	*	—	—	1	—	5	4	3	15	8	/	—	10	—	7	8	8
Family planning nurse	1	1	2	—	—	—	3	2	2	3	2	4	—	2	—	9	4	2
Number of nurses (= 100%)	824	457	171	132	64	609	291	371	102	1057	67	442	42	221	136	44	50	52

3 Work organisation

This chapter looks at some aspects of nurses work organisation, for example the extent of full, part-time and relief work, relationships with general practice in terms of attachment and number of practices worked with and the amount of clerical and clinical support available to nurses working in the community.

3.1 Full, part-time and relief working

Nurses were asked the number of hours they worked in a week.† Their answers will be discussed in detail in Chapter 7 in conjunction with information from the diaries. In Table 3.1 the proportions working full and part-time are given—part-time work being 30 hours or less per week. The table shows at one extreme that only 2% of community psychiatric nurses worked part-time but this applied to 95% of family planning nurses. Just under a fifth of both district nurses and health visitors were part-time whereas the majority of auxiliaries and GP employed practice nurses worked part-time. Among district nurses those with a district nursing qualification

were much less likely to be part-timers than those who did not have district training.

These differences in hours worked are reflected in the answers to the next question—'On how many days (nights) a week do you normally work (excluding 'on call' days)'—shown in Table 3.2. Again family planning nurses stand out from the others in that one quarter of them worked on only one day; only one tenth worked on five days each week. The majority of all other types of nurses worked on five days a week. This suggests that many of the part-time nurses worked short hours on each day of the week rather than full-time hours on only some days of the week.

All nurses were asked a short series of questions† about the extent of relief working. The answers to these have been combined and are shown at Table 3.3. At the first

---

†Question 13 How many hours on average do you work in a week (excluding 'on call' time)?

†Q4 Apart from your main work do you do any relief work?
If YES—(a) Do you do covering or relief work as part of formal arrangements . . . . . or informally for colleagues?
(b) Thinking about the last month, what proportion of your working and on call time was spent doing relief work?

Table 3.1 Full and part-time working, by type of nurse

	All DNs	DN SRN+	DN SRN −	DN SEN+	DN SEN −	Auxil-iaries	GP empl.	Mid-wives	DN/ Midw.	HV	HV ass.	Schl. Nurse	Sch.N ass.	Fam. Plan.	Comm. Psych.	Geri-atric	Liai-son	Clinic
	%	%	%	%	%	%	%	%	%	%	%	%	%	%	%	%	%	%
Part-time	18	10	46	6	25	67	74	10	5	17	57	49	16	95	2	27	14	52
Full-time	82	90	54	94	75	33	26	90	95	83	43	51	84	5	98	73	86	48
Number of nurses (= 100%)	824	457	171	132	64	609	291	371	102	1057	67	442	42	221	136	44	50	52

Table 3.2 Number of days worked per week, by type of nurse

Number of days on which work is normally done per week	All DNs	DN SRN+	DN SRN −	DN SEN+	DN SEN −	Auxil-iaries	GP empl.	Mid-wives	DN/ Midw.	HV	HV ass.	Schl. Nurse	Sch.N ass.	Fam. Plan.	Comm. Psych.	Geri-atric	Liai-son	Clinic
	%	%	%	%	%	%	%	%	%	%	%	%	%	%	%	%	%	%
One	*	*	2	—	—	1	2	*	—	*	1	*	—	26	—	—	—	2
Two	4	2	14	—	1	7	6	1	1	1	5	1	—	27	—	2	2	2
Three	5	4	9	—	6	8	9	1	2	6	15	6	5	26	1	14	2	16
Four	3	2	5	3	7	6	19	2	—	8	18	14	3	12	3	2	6	14
Five	87	91	69	95	86	78	57	95	96	85	61	79	92	9	94	82	90	64
Six	1	1	1	2	—	*	7	1	1	*	—	*	—	*	1	—	—	2
Seven	*	*	*	—	—	*	*	—	—	—	—	*	—	—	1	—	—	—
Number of nurses (= 100%)	824	457	171	132	64	609	291	371	102	1057	67	442	42	216	136	44	50	52

Table 3.3 Amounts of formal and informal relief work carried out, by type of nurse

Amount of relief work	All DNs	DN SRN+	DN SRN −	DN SEN+	DN SEN −	Auxil-iaries	GP empl.	Mid-wives	DN/ Midw.	HV	HV ass.	Schl. Nurse	Sch.N ass.	Fam. Plan.	Comm. Psych.	Geri-atric	Liai-son	Clinic
	%	%	%	%	%	%	%	%	%	%	%	%	%	%	%	%	%	%
Full-time relief nurse	10	6	23	10	8	2	*	4	6	1	—	*	—	*	—	5	—	2
½ time or more – formal	4 } 5	4 } 4	* } *	3 } 5	4 } 5	1 } 1	1 } 1	6 } 9	7 } 7	1 } *	*	*	—	1 } 2	— } 2	2 } 2	2 } 2	4 } 4
– informal	1	*	*	2	1	1	1	3	—	*				1	2	2	2	2
¼ < ½ time – formal	8 } 9	8 } 10	6 } 7	9 } 11	6 } 8	1 } 2	1 } 24	19 } 24	18 } 25	2 } 4	5 } 8	2 } 3	—	3 } 6	4 } 6	3 } 5	2 } 4	2 } 2
– informal	1	2	1	2	2	1	2	5	7	2	3	1		3	2	2	2	
Less than ¼ – formal	16 } 26	19 } 31	11 } 19	16 } 26	7 } 11	12 } 18	8 } 17	15 } 22	23 } 31	15 } 32	20 } 40	21 } 33	21 } 33	19 } 40	7 } 22	11 } 18	8 } 14	21 } 31
– informal	10	12	8	10	4	6	9	7	8	17	20	12	12	21	15	7	6	10
No relief work	50	49	47	50	68	77	80	41	31	62	52	64	67	52	70	75	82	61
Number of nurses (= 100%)	824	457	171	132	64	609	291	371	102	1057	67	442	42	221	136	44	50	52

part of the question a small proportion of the nurses identified themselves as full-time relief nurses. These were often known as 'bank nurses'. Formal arrangements for relief work were generally more common than informal arrangements, especially where the proportion of time spent doing relief duty was a quarter or more of the last month's work. Relief duty for most nurses who did any took up less than quarter of their time. The majority of all nurses except district nurses, midwives and joint duty staff did no relief work at all. Among district nurses almost one quarter of the SRNs without district training were full-time relief nurses.

3.2 Attachment and geographical patch working

Attachment or alignment are formal arrangements under which community nursing staff are responsible for providing services to people on lists of specified GPs. Specialist nurses are not normally attached to general practices as it is not appropriate to organise their work in that way. Only the main types of nurses, therefore, were asked about attachment† and working with GPs— obviously GP employed practice nurses were not asked about attachment.

Table 3.4 shows the proportions of these nurses with different patterns of attachment and patch working. The base numbers are smaller than on previous tables because full-time relief nurses were not asked about attachment, so they are not included in the 'district nurses' or 'auxiliaries' categories on this table. Over 80% of district nurses, midwives and health visitors were attached to general practices. The proportion was smaller (68%) but still substantial for auxiliaries and health visitor assistants. Most of the nurses who were not attached worked entirely on a geographical patch system. Eight per

cent of auxiliaries had their work organised in other ways— they either worked from a clinic, hospital or centre or were allocated work by a supervisor or the Area Health Authority.

Table 3.3 shows that a high proportion, 23%, of district nurse SRNs without district training were relief nurses. Having excluded these from Table 3.4 it can be seen that compared with other district nurses, this group were also less likely to be attached to general practice.

Four different working arrangements among attached nurses were identified at the pilot stage of the survey, the main one being where the nurse cared for patients in all parts of the GP's catchment area. Some nurses cared for patients in specific parts of the GP's area implying that the list had been divided up on a geographical basis and shared between staff. The third and fourth types of arrangements were where nurses cared for people on GP lists but also had responsibilites for patients in a geographical patch regardless of their GP.†

As can be seen from Table 3.4 the full type of attachment was most common for each of the groups of staff. Almost one half of all district nurses and auxiliaries were attached and cared for patients in all parts of a GP's area. A further 12% of them worked in part of a catchment area only. Health visitors were more likely than district nurses to work in only a part of a catchment area. A quarter of both types of staff had responsibilities for a patch in addition to the patients on their attached GP's list. Midwives and joint duty staff were even more likely than district nurses and health visitors to have a patch in addition to their attachment—44% of them did. So even though the vast majority of these main types of community nurses had formal attachments to general practice many worked in only a part of the GP's catchment area and/or had an additional geographical patch.

These working arrangements are reflected in the numbers of GPs and practices that nurses worked with. This is considered next in relation to all the staff including those who were not formally attached to general practice.

---

†Q5. I'd now like to read a definition to you—
'Attachment or alignment are formal arrangements under which staff are responsible for providing services to people on the lists of specified general practitioners'.
(Apart from any relief work) Are you attached or aligned to general practitioners in this way at all?
If no
(a) May I just check—Does that mean you work a geographical patch only?
If no
(b) So you are neither formally attached or aligned and you do not work entirely on a geographical patch system, how then is your work organised?

---

†Q6 Do you care for patients in all parts of the GP's catchment area or only those who live in specific parts?
Q7 Do you care only for people on specific GP lists or are you responsible for an additional geographical patch?

Table 3.4 Patterns of attachment and patch working, by type of nurse

Working patterns	All DNs	DN SRN+	DN SRN –	DN SEN+	DN SEN –	Auxil- iaries	Mid- wives	DN/ Midw.	HV	HV ass.
	%	%	%	%	%	%	%	%	%	%
Not attached – works patch only	16	14	32	5	18	24	17	11	10	18
Not attached – other†	1	1	3	—	5	8	2	—	1	9
Attached and covers										
all parts of GP area	47	46	42	62	35	45	33	30	37	54
specific areas only	12	15	5	7	11	12	5	16	27	12
	} 83	} 85	} 65	} 95	} 77	} 68	} 83	} 89	} 89	} 73
all parts plus patch	15	15	13	14	15	7	28	24	12	7
specific areas plus patch	9	9	5	12	16	4	15	19	13	—
*Number of nurses (= 100%)†† *	732	427	129	117	59	517	350	94	1039	67

†These nurses did not work a patch system, neither were they attached. They had their work organised in other ways eg from a clinic, hospital or centre or were allocated work by a supervisor or the Area Health Authority.

††Base numbers are smaller than on previous tables because full-time relief nurses, night sitters and bath attendants were excluded.

Table 3.5 shows the proportions of nurses who worked with different numbers of GPs. For all types of nurses the majority worked with four or more GPs. Midwives tended to work with a large number of GPs—55% of midwives worked with seven or more. This was not the case for district nurse/midwives as only 27% worked with seven or more GPs.

Health visitors worked with smaller numbers of GPs—34% of them worked with two or three. Auxiliaries and health visitor assistants were the only type of staff with an appreciable proportion who had no contact with GPs. GP employed practice nurses were asked about the GPs they worked with. Forty-three per cent worked with less than four GPs.

Table 3.6 shows the number of different practices involved. As one would expect, 95% of GP employed practice nurses worked with only one practice. Over one half of the health visitors and district nurse/midwives worked with only one practice and just under half (47%)

of the district nurses. Midwives were the only type of nurse where the largest proportion were not working with only one practice—only 20% of them did. Just over one quarter of midwives worked with five or more practices.

Nurses were asked whether the GPs they worked with worked in a health centre or in their own practice premises. Table 3.7 shows that the majority of GPs worked with were in their own premises. However, between one third and one half of district nurses, midwives, health visitors and auxiliaries worked with GPs in health centres. Only 17% of GP employed nurses worked in health centres.

3.3 Work base, office and clerical support

As can be seen from Table 3.8 there was a large variation between different types of nurses in the place from which they worked on a daily basis.* More than 80% of midwives and joint duty district nurse/midwives worked

*Q17 Where do you work from on a daily basis?

Table 3.5 Number of general practitioners (GPs) worked with, by type of nurse

Number of GPs worked with	All DNs	DN SRN+	DN SRN −	DN SEN+	DN SEN −	Auxiliaries	GP empl.	Mid-wives	DN/Midw.	HV	HV ass.
	%	%	%	%	%	%	%	%	%	%	%
One	1	2	1	1	2	1	10	2	2	4	2
Two	8	8	8	5	12	8	16	5	9	15	6
Three	14	16	8	9	20	10	17	5	23	19	18
Four to six	42	40	42	54	32	40	46	32	39	39	31
Seven to ten	15	16	8	21	16	19	10	25	15	12	17
More than ten	18	17	29	10	15	10	1	30	12	9	12
None – no GP contact	2	1	4	—	3	12	—	1	—	2	14
Number of nurses (= 100%)†	*824*	*457*	*171*	*132*	*64*	*609*	*291*	*346*	*94*	*1039*	*67*

†Base numbers are smaller than on previous tables because full-time relief nurses, night sitters and bath attendants were excluded.

Table 3.6 Number of practices worked with, by type of nurse

Number of practices worked with	All DNs	DN SRN+	DN SRN −	DN SEN+	DN SEN −	Auxiliaries	GP empl.	Mid-wives	DN/Midw.	HV	HV ass.
	%	%	%	%	%	%	%	%	%	%	%
One	46	49	36	46	52	36	95	20	55	60	33
Two	20	20	12	30	15	19	3	26	15	19	26
Three	9	10	11	7	5	12	2	18	8	5	14
Four	5	4	6	3	10	8	*	7	7	3	5
Five or more	17	16	25	13	13	11	—	27	15	11	5
Don't know	1	*	6	1	2	2	—	1	—	*	3
No contact with GPs	2	1	4	—	3	12	—	1	—	2	14
Number of nurses (= 100%)†	*732*	*426*	*129*	*117*	*59*	*517*	*291*	*346*	*94*	*1039*	*67*

†Base numbers are smaller than on previous tables because full-time relief nurses, night sitters and bath attendants were excluded.

Table 3.7 Working base of GPs with whom nurses work, by type of nurse

Working base of GPs worked with	All DNs	DN SRN+	DN SRN −	DN SEN+	DN SEN −	Auxiliaries	GP empl.	Mid-wives	DN/Midw.	HV	HV ass.
	%	%	%	%	%	%	%	%	%	%	%
Own practice premises	60	62	52	62	57	48	82	49	81	65	42
Health centre	14	15	9	13	20	16	9	10	4	15	18
Own practice premises and health centre	23	21	34	24	18	22	8	40	15	18	23
Don't know	1	1	1	1	2	2	1	*	—	*	3
No contact with GPs	2	1	4	—	3	12	—	1	—	2	14
Number of nurses (= 100%)†	*824*	*457*	*171*	*132*	*64*	*609*	*291*	*346*	*94*	*1039*	*67*

†Base numbers are smaller than on previous tables because full-time relief nurses, night sitters and bath attendants were excluded.

from home. Three fifths of district nurses and two thirds of auxiliaries were based at home as were one fifth of geriatric and liaison nurses. Among district nurses those with district training were more likely to be based at home than those without. Only a small proportion of the other types of nurses worked from home. Not surprisingly 81% of community psychiatric nurses were based in a hospital and 95% of GP employed nurses worked from practice premises or a health centre. The large majority of health visitors, school nurses, family planning and clinic nurses worked from clinics or health centres. Very few nurses working in the community (apart from those employed by GPs) worked from practice premises.

The pilot survey found that most nurses who worked from home regarded their home as their office. Those who did not work from home were asked, 'Do you have your own office, shared office space or no office?' Their answers are shown in Table 3.9. Few nurses had access to their own office although in general most of those who did not work from home had shared office space. This was not true for family planning nurses, one half of whom had no office.

Those groups of staff—district nurses, midwives and joint duty staff—who were traditionally based at home were also much less likely than other types of nurse to have staff to call on to help with clerical work.† Table 3.10 shows that only five per cent of midwives and two per cent

of joint duty staff had access to clerical support. Somewhat more, 15% of district nurses had some clerical support, but between one half and two thirds of health visitors, GP nurses, school, family planning, community psychiatric and clinic nurses could call on help with their clerical work.

3.4 Clinical support

Table 3.11 shows that the majority of all types of nurses had 'access to a treatment or interview room where they could see clients/patients in private'.†† However a higher proportion of health visitors and school nurses than of district nurses or midwives had such a facility, 88% compared with 61% of district nurses and 65% of midwives.

Another aspect of clinical work that was asked about was whether the nurse had any 'staff that you personally can call on for assistance with clinical work'.††† Answers are given in Table 3.12 where it can be seen that staff working in the district nursing service, district nurses and joint duty staff, were much more likely than other nurses to have auxiliaries and assistants available to help them. Three fifths had this kind of support. About one third of

†Q21 Do you have any staff you can call on for assistance with clerical work?
††Q19 Do you have any access ...?
†††Q20 Apart from relief work, do you have any staff ...?

Table 3.8 Work base, by type of nurse

Work base	All DNs	DN SRN+	DN SRN –	DN SEN+	DN SEN –	Auxil-iaries	GP empl.	Mid-wives	DN/ Midw.	HV	HV ass.	Schl. Nurse	Sch.N ass.	Fam. Plan.	Comm. Psych.	Geria-tric	Liai-son	Clinic
	%	%	%	%	%	%	%	%	%	%	%	%	%	%	%	%	%	%
Home	61	64	51	72	49	67	3	88	84	6	7	13	14	9	4	20	22	4
Clinic	8	6	11	6	15	12	1	2	10	44	36	40	45	56	5	34	10	23
Health centre	15	16	16	11	21	12	10	3	2	35	47	30	17	25	6	30	16	57
Practice premises	4	5	3	3	5	3	85	1	4	9	7	—	—	1	—	9	2	6
Hospital	5	4	9	2	4	2	—	6	—	2	—	*	—	5	81	5	44	8
Community health office	3	2	6	2	1	2	—	—	—	3	3	3	10	—	—	—	—	2
School	—	—	—	—	—	*	—	—	—	—	—	12	12	—	—	—	—	—
Other	4	3	4	4	5	2	1	—	—	1	—	2	2	4	4	2	6	—
Number of nurses (= 100%)	824	457	171	132	64	609	291	371	102	1057	67	442	42	221	136	44	50	52

Table 3.9 Access to office space, by type of nurse

Access to office space	All DNs	DN SRN+	DN SRN –	DN SEN+	DN SEN –	Auxil-iaries	GP empl.	Mid-wives	DN/ Midw.	HV	HV ass.	Schl. Nurse	Sch.N ass.	Fam. Plan.	Comm. Psych.	Geria-tric	Liai-son	Clinic
	%	%	%	%	%	%	%	%	%	%	%	%	%	%	%	%	%	%
Own office	2	2	4	—	—	*	31	1	—	10	3	14	—	13	9	7	8	15
Shared office	28	26	33	24	36	16	47	6	8	83	85	65	72	28	85	71	68	66
No office	9	8	12	4	15	17	19	5	8	1	5	8	14	50	2	2	2	15
Works from home	61	64	51	72	49	67	3	88	84	6	7	13	14	9	4	20	22	4
Number of nurses (= 100%)	824	457	171	132	64	609	291	371	102	1057	67	442	42	221	136	44	50	52

Table 3.10 Assistance with clerical work, by type of nurse

Assistance with clerical work	All DNs	DN SRN+	DN SRN –	DN SEN+	DN SEN –	GP empl.	Mid-wives	DN/ Midw.	HV	Schl. Nurse	Fam. Plan.	Comm. Psych.	Geria-tric	Liai-son	Clinic
	%	%	%	%	%	%	%	%	%	%	%	%	%	%	%
Yes	15	12	14	20	31	67	5	2	57	49	68	60	32	35	51
No	85	88	86	80	69	33	95	98	43	51	32	40	68	65	49
Number of nurses (= 100%)†	732	427	129	117	59	291	350	94	1039	441	221	136	44	50	52

†Some of the bases are smaller than on previous tables because full-time relief nurses were not asked this question.

Table 3.11 Access to treatment or interview room, by type of nurse

Access to treatment room	All DNs	DN SRN+	DN SRN –	DN SEN+	DN SEN –	GP empl.	Mid-wives	DN/ Midw.	HV	HV ass.	Schl. Nurse	Sch.N ass.	Fam. Plan.	Comm. Psych.	Geria-tric	Liai-son	Clinic
	%	%	%	%	%	%	%	%	%	%	%	%	%	%	%	%	%
Yes	61	67	45	63	64	96	65	70	88	84	88	76	96	77	79	68	82
No	39	33	55	37	36	4	35	30	12	16	12	24	4	23	21	32	18
Number of nurses (= 100%)	824	457	171	132	64	291	371	102	1057	67	442	42	221	136	44	50	52

health visitors, school, psychiatric and clinic nurses could call on clinical assistance.

3.5 Attachment and clinical and clerical support

Table 3.13 presents the proportions of nurses with access to a treatment room, clinical assistance, their own or shared office space and clerical support. Auxiliaries are excluded from this table because the questions were not relevant to them.

District nurses
Access to a treatment room and clinical assistance was better for attached district nurses than for the not attached; for example, 70% of attached nurses had access to a treatment room compared with 28% of not attached district nurses. In addition those who worked in GP catchment areas only were rather better off than those who worked an additional patch. A large proportion of district nurses were based in their own homes but this was less common among the not attached. Forty-four per cent

of them had their own or shared office space compared with 28% of attached staff. Access to help with clerical work was not related to attachment patterns.

Midwives
There were no statistically significant differences between the various groups of midwives for any of these four aspects of their working situation.

Health visitors
There was no difference between the various groups of health visitors except that the not attached more often had assistance with their clinical work than the attached, 47% compared with 31%.

In general therefore attachment or different attachment arrangements appeared to be unrelated to these four aspects of nurses' working situations for health visitors or midwives. But attached district nurses reported better clinical support in terms of treatment rooms and assistance than not attached district nurses.

Table 3.12 Whether able to call on assistance for clinical work, by type of nurse

Assistance with clinical work	All DNs	DN SRN+	DN SRN −	DN SEN+	DN SEN −	GP empl.	Mid- wives	DN/ Midw.	HV	Schl. Nurse	Fam. Plan	Comm. Psych.	Geria- tric	Liai- son	Clinic
	%	%	%	%	%	%	%	%	%	%	%	%	%	%	%
Yes	59	65	50	56	46	10	17	60	33	30	8	31	23	7	33
No	41	35	50	44	54	90	83	40	67	70	92	69	77	93	67
Number of nurses (= 100%)†	732	427	129	117	59	291	350	94	1039	441	221	136	44	50	52

†Some of the bases are smaller than on previous tables because full-time relief nurses were not asked this question.

Table 3.13 Clinical and clerical support, by type of attachment

Proportion with access to:	Not attached	Attached		Attached		
		All parts	Specific parts	All + patch	Specific + patch	All attached
District nurses	%	%	%	%	%	%
treatment room	28	73	73	57	67	70
clinical assistance	45	64	67	58	58	63
office space	44	24	35	31	31	28
clerical support	12	13	11	26	15	15
Number of district nurses (= 100%)	126	336	87	105	66	594
Midwives	%	%		%	%	%
treatment room	55	71	(13)	70	52	67
clinical assistance	20	18	(3)	14	15	16
office space	9	6	(0)	10	2	6
clerical support	6	4	(1)	3	9	5
Number of midwives (= 100%)	66	114	18	97	54	283
Health visitors	%	%	%	%	%	%
treatment room	89	87	89	84	94	88
clinical assistance	47	33	26	40	31	31
office space	93	93	93	95	96	94
clerical support	50	64	55	52	53	58
Number of health visitors (= 100%)	120	380	282	120	132	914

Auxiliaries were not asked these questions.

4 Opinions on client/patient related issues

At the pilot stage of the survey nurses were asked—'If you had more time, are there particular aspects of your job that you would like to spend some time or more time on?' If yes—'What particular aspects of your job would you like to spend more time on?' There was great interest in this question among the nurses interviewed and from these answers three different areas were chosen for special questions at the main stage of the survey—client groups, counselling and clinics. The answers to these are described in this chapter together with responses to questions about client/patient care.

4.1 Groups of clients/patients in need of more care

Nurses were asked whether 'in your opinion ... there are particular groups of clients/patients in your district that are in need of more care from nurses working in the community?' From the answers given to this question at the pilot stage of the survey a list of 14 client groups was devised which was handed to nurses to help them answer. Many nurses gave more than one answer to the question and were then asked 'which group, of those you have mentioned, do you think is *most* in need of more care from nurses working in the community?' By combining the answers to the first part of the question from those who gave only one group and from the second part of the question for those initially giving more than one group, one priority group was identified for each nurse. Table 4.1 shows which groups were regarded by the different types of nurses as most in need of more community nursing care.

As can be seen the elderly (the elderly living alone and the elderly generally) were mentioned more often than any other client group. This was true for all types of nurses including school and family planning nurses whose work did not generally include care of the elderly. District nurses, geriatric and liaison nurses more often than other types of nurses said that the elderly were most in need of more care. They were followed closely by other staff working in the district nursing service—joint duty staff and auxiliaries, three fifths of whom regarded the elderly as the priority group. Fifty-two per cent of GP employed nurses felt the elderly were most in need as did 43% of health visitors.

Most of the client groups on the list presented to respondents were singled out by fewer than ten per cent of any of the different types of nurses. However significant minorities of midwives, joint duty staff and health visitors mentioned pregnant women or mothers with new babies. Fifteen per cent of district and 18% of geriatric nurses mentioned the terminally ill. Not surprisingly 40% of community psychiatric nurses regarded the mentally handicapped or the mentally ill as being the priority group of patients for more community nursing care.

4.2 Groups of clients/patients on whom nurses would like to spend more time

This question—'If you had more time, are there any particular groups of clients/patients that you would like to spend some time, or more time on?'—was asked and the priority group identified in the same way as the question discussed previously. The client groups that nurses would *most* like to spend more time on are shown in Table 4.2. This table therefore reflects the nurses' *personal* views on the groups that they would like to spend some or more time with. The replies did not necessarily relate to the client groups that nurses dealt with as part of their current job—a particular school nurse, for instance, might want to spend time on the elderly even though she did not spend any time on them at all in her current school nursing job.

Table 4.1 Groups of clients/patients thought to be most in need of more care from nurses working in the community, by type of nurse

Client group	All DNs	DN SRN+	DN SRN –	DN SEN+	DN SEN –	Auxil-iaries	GP empl.	Mid-wives	DN/midw.	HV	HV ass.	Schl. Nurse	Sch.N ass.	Fam. Plan.	Comm. Psych.	Geria-tric	Liai-son	Clinic
	%	%	%	%	%	%	%	%	%	%	%	%	%	%	%	%	%	%
Pregnant women	*	*	*	—	—	—	1	12	9	8	—	1	—	2	—	—	2	—
Mothers and new babies	*	*	*	—	1	1	4	14	3	7	—	1	—	8	1	—	2	2
Under fives	*	—	*	—	—	*	1	1	—	5	3	2	2	2	1	—	2	—
School children	—	—	—	—	—	*	1	—	—	1	1	9	—	3	1	—	—	2
One parent families	—	—	—	—	—	*	2	11	2	5	—	9	7	7	2	—	—	—
Elderly living alone	44	44	47	42	39	42	29	14	40	23	52	24	20	23	16	48	48	39
Elderly (generally)	19	18	22	15	23	13	23	4	15	20	18	9	20	5	17	18	14	6
Mentally handicapped	1	1	1	2	1	1	—	1	—	3	—	5	10	4	10	—	4	—
Physically handicapped	3	3	2	4	1	3	*	1	2	2	1	3	—	1	—	5	—	2
Mentally ill	2	2	1	3	—	1	3	3	1	3	8	3	2	—	2	30	5	2
Terminally ill	15	14	13	20	17	5	4	3	6	3	6	3	7	5	—	18	2	11
Post operative/hospital discharge	1	1	1	1	1	1	2	1	2	1	—	1	5	4	2	2	6	2
Ethnic minorities	—	—	—	—	—	—	*	6	1	2	—	2	—	5	—	—	—	2
Relatives of clients	2	2	*	2	1	2	2	—	—	2	—	3	—	1	12	7	4	2
Other	1	1	*	—	2	*	1	2	1	2	2	3	2	4	7	2	6	—
None	12	14	12	11	14	31	27	29	16	8	14	23	27	24	2	2	8	32
Number of nurses (= 100%)	824	457	171	132	64	609	291	371	102	1057	67	442	42	221	136	44	50	52

Those working in the district nursing service, GP nurses, geriatric and liaison nurses again all said that they would choose to spend more time with the elderly than with any group of patients. In Table 4.1 health visitors mentioned the elderly as being most in need of community nursing care more frequently than their traditional client groups of pregnant women and mothers with babies and children under five. However when asked how they would like to spend some hypothetical extra time more of them chose mothers and young children (41%) than chose the elderly (24%).

4.3 Areas of counselling and health education on which nurses would like to spend more time

Nurses working in the community are important providers of advice and health education to clients/patients in the community. It was also an area of work that nurses in the pilot survey frequently expressed a wish to spend more time on. The majority of all types of nurses except school nurse assistants and clinic nurses said they would like to do more counselling and health education.† Nurses were handed a card with a list of topic areas and asked to choose which one they would like to spend more time on. Their answers are shown in Table 4.3.

†Q27 If you had more time, would you like to do more counselling and health education? If yes a) which particular area would you like to spend more time on? b) Which area, of those you have mentioned, would you *most* like to spend more time on?

For each type of nurse there were one or two topic areas that were more frequently mentioned than others. For example district nurses and geriatric nurses singled out physical health; midwives and joint duty staff pregnancy, labour and childcare. Health visitors most frequently mentioned childcare and health education in schools as also did school nurses. Family planning nurses most often wanted to spend more counselling time on family planning and marital and psychosexual problems. The latter were also mentioned fairly frequently by community psychiatric nurses whose primary concern was mental health problems.

4.4 Types of clinics on which nurses would like to spend more time

Again when asked 'What about clinics, would you like to extend this aspect of your work if you had the time?' the majority of all types of nurses except liaison and clinic nurses said they would. They were then handed a card listing different kinds of clinics. The type of clinics they wanted most to spend more time on are shown at Table 4.4.

More than one fifth of district nurses wanted most to spend more time in GP surgery sessions, a further tenth named well woman or cytology clinics. Ante/post natal clinics were most popular among midwifery staff. Rather similar proportions of health visitors mentioned each of ante/post natal, infant welfare, developmental

Table 4.2 Groups of clients/patients nurses would most like to spend more time on, by type of nurse

Client type	All DNs	DN SRN+	DN SRN −	DN SEN+	DN SEN −	GP empl.	Mid-wives	DN/ Midw.	HV	HV ass.	Schl. Nurse	Sch.N ass.	Fam. Plan.	Comm. Psych.	Geria-tric	Liai-son	Clinic
	%	%	%	%	%	%	%	%	%	%	%	%	%	%	%	%	%
Pregnant women	1	1	1	—	1	5	32	22	20	—	—	—	6	1	—	—	—
Mothers and new babies	1	1	2	1	1	14	30	14	11	4	2	5	15	2	—	4	15
Under fives	*	*	*	—	1	1	—	—	10	3	9	10	—	2	2	—	13
School children	*	—	—	2	—	2	2	—	5	9	29	19	9	4	—	6	2
One parent families	*	1	—	—	—	2	7	—	5	—	5	3	4	5	—	—	—
Elderly living alone	28	25	32	30	35	9	2	29	11	30	9	3	4	12	37	23	4
Elderly (generally)	15	15	13	18	19	17	1	11	13	22	5	3	3	5	14	12	11
Mentally handicapped	1	*	1	1	—	1	*	1	2	2	3	3	1	3	2	—	2
Physically handicapped	6	7	4	5	4	1	*	1	3	3	4	—	2	—	14	2	—
Mentally ill	1	1	2	1	2	3	—	—	1	2	1	—	—	36	—	—	2
Terminally ill	28	29	27	28	20	5	1	8	2	9	1	—	3	—	4	6	—
Post operative/hospital discharge	2	2	2	1	—	3	—	—	1	1	*	3	*	1	—	4	4
Ethnic minorities	*	*	*	—	2	*	4	—	2	—	2	—	4	1	—	6	—
Relatives of clients	4	4	3	4	3	2	1	3	2	2	5	—	1	14	9	6	2
Other	3	4	2	1	3	4	3	4	5	3	3	—	13	10	4	12	2
None	10	10	11	8	9	31	17	7	7	10	22	51	35	4	14	19	43
Number of nurses (= 100%)	*824*	*457*	*171*	*132*	*64*	*291*	*371*	*102*	*1057*	*67*	*442*	*42*	*221*	*136*	*44*	*50*	*52*

Table 4.3 Areas for counselling and health education nurses would most like to spend more time on, by type of nurse

Topic areas	All DNs	DN SRN+	DN SRN −	DN SEN+	DN SEN −	GP empl.	Mid-wives	DN/ Midw.	HV	HV ass.	Schl. Nurse	Sch.N ass.	Fam. Plan.	Comm. Psych.	Geria-tric	Liai-son	Clinic
	%	%	%	%	%	%	%	%	%	%	%	%	%	%	%	%	%
Pregnancy and labour	1	1	1	—	2	2	24	29	6	—	*	—	4	1	2	—	2
Nutrition†	2	2	2	2	—	3	10	2	6	—	*	—	1	—	—	4	—
Child care††	3	2	4	4	6	12	16	12	31	9	10	5	3	6	4	6	6
Immunisation and vaccination	2	2	1	4	2	8	*	1	*	12	1	—	—	—	—	2	8
Family planning	5	5	5	4	2	11	7	8	3	3	3	3	20	—	5	2	4
Marital and psychosexual	2	2	4	—	2	4	3	1	8	—	2	—	27	13	4	6	2
Physical health	27	29	26	23	21	6	*	9	2	9	1	—	1	1	30	16	4
Mental health	5	4	6	8	5	5	1	—	3	5	1	3	1	54	5	2	—
Health education in schools	5	4	9	5	8	8	7	7	17	16	48	6	13	9	4	6	11
Other†††	7	7	8	4	3	2	1	2	2	3	3	—	2	1	14	28	7
None	41	42	34	46	49	39	31	29	22	43	31	83	28	15	32	28	56
Number of nurses (= 100%)	*824*	*457*	*171*	*132*	*64*	*291*	*371*	*102*	*1057*	*67*	*442*	*42*	*221*	*136*	*44*	*50*	*52*

†Nutrition including infant feeding.
††Child care/child development/parentcraft.
†††This category largely consisted of topic areas relating to the elderly, bereavement and terminal illness.

assessment and parentcraft. One quarter of family planning clinic nurses chose well woman or cytology clinics—this was a greater proportion than would choose to spend more time doing family planning. Community psychiatric, geriatric and liaison nurses gave large numbers of answers that fell into the 'other' category. These were largely referring to clinics specifically to help the mentally ill and elderly.

4.5 Assessment of various aspects of client/patient care

Nurses were asked about six aspects of client/patient care as part of a composite question containing eight separate questions†. The two relating to relationships with GPs are discussed in Chapter 5. Nurses were asked to assess aspects of their work using a five point scale from very good to very poor. The full answers to the six questions about client/patient care are given in the appendix to this chapter but Table 4.5 summarises these by giving the proportions who made assessments of very good or good.

The question was posed six times with the aspects of care presented in alphabetical order. However in the table they are ranked in the order in which the total (weighted) sample of nurses rated them. So for example it can be seen that 'knowledge of the geographical area worked in' was generally rated higher than 'the opportunity to get to know clients/patients' and 'the opportunity to get to know clients'/patients' familes' was generally rated the lowest of these six aspects of care.

†Q32 How would you assess the following things in your current work? (a-h see Table 4.5.) Please choose the answers from the card—very good, good, fair, poor, very poor.

Knowledge of the geographical area was rated highly by all types of nurses except GP nurses, family planning and clinic nurses. Large proportions of these nurses made no visits as part of their work.

Many types of nurses rated the 'quality of client/patient care' equal or better than 'the opportunity to get to know clients/patients'. However, a very large group of staff—health visitors—assessed the 'quality of care' as less good than 'the opportunity to get to know clients'.

Some 99% of GP employed nurses rated access to patients' records as very good or good. Only just over 70% of district nurses and joint duty staff rated access this highly although just over 80% of midwives and health visitors felt that it was very good or good. Of the specialist nurses geriatric nurses seemed to be at a particular disadvantage in relation to access to patients' records.

Continuity of care was generally assessed to be less good than quality of care. Again, as with quality, health visitors rated it lower than district nurses, midwives and GP nurses.

The opportunity to get to know clients'/patients' families was rated markedly lower than other aspects of patient care by assistant and GP employed nurses and by all types of specialist nurses except community psychiatric staff, 77% of whom rated it as very good or good. This was also true for district nurse SRNs without district training. Their assessments were lower than those of other district nurses on all these questions—a reflection of the high proportions who were relief or part-time staff.

Table 4.4 Type of clinics that nurses would most like to spend more time on, by type of nurse

Type of clinic	All DNs	DN SRN+	DN SRN −	DN SEN+	DN SEN −	GP empl.	Mid-wives	DN/ Midw.	HV	HV ass.	Schl. Nurse	Sch.N ass.	Fam. Plan.	Comm. Psych.	Geria-tric	Liai-son	Clinic
	%	%	%	%	%	%	%	%	%	%	%	%	%	%	%	%	%
Ante/post natal†	1	1	1	1	1	5	32	23	9	1	1	—	5	4	—	4	2
Infant welfare††	2	1	4	4	5	5	2	2	10	15	8	18	1	—	—	2	11
Development assessment	1	*	2	2	—	2	2	—	15	5	12	—	*	9	2	2	2
Immunisation and vaccination	2	2	1	2	2	4	—	1	*	5	1	—	—	—	—	—	6
Parentcraft/mothercraft	1	1	1	—	—	4	11	5	10	—	1	2	1	3	—	—	—
Family planning	5	4	6	6	5	8	5	9	3	6	4	3	18	—	2	—	—
Well woman, cytology	12	13	9	12	7	17	4	10	5	12	4	—	25	—	—	2	11
Hearing and vision	1	1	2	2	2	2	—	2	1	5	6	—	—	—	3	4	2
School medicals	1	—	2	—	5	2	—	—	*	1	9	16	—	—	—	—	2
GP surgery sessions	22	20	23	23	26	4	3	4	4	1	*	—	6	18	10	8	4
Slimming/obesity	4	5	5	3	2	6	1	2	3	1	7	3	3	1	2	2	6
Blood pressure	6	7	4	8	*	9	*	5	1	8	1	—	1	2	19	2	—
Other	3	4	3	1	2	1	—	3	4	3	2	—	4	31	24	16	4
None	39	41	37	36	43	31	40	29	35	37	44	58	36	32	38	58	50
Number of nurses (= 100%)	824	457	171	132	64	291	371	102	1057	67	442	42	221	136	44	50	52

†Includes antenatal, postnatal, relaxation, psychoprophylaxis.
††Includes well baby, infant welfare, child health.

Table 4.5 Summary table* showing proportions rating as very good or good† various aspects of client/patient care, by type of nurse.

Assessment of:	All DNs	DN SRN+	DN SRN −	DN SEN+	DN SEN −	GP empl.	Mid-wives	DN/ Midw.	HV	HV ass.	Schl. Nurse	Sch.N ass.	Fam. Plan.	Comm. Psych.	Geria-tric	Liai-son	Clinic
(h) knowledge of the geographical area worked in	93%	96%	81%	98%	86%	58%	93%	88%	91%	85%	88%	90%	54%	85%	95%	92%	50%
(a) opportunity to get to know clients/patients	89%	92%	82%	86%	86%	87%	81%	88%	87%	79%	76%	74%	74%	92%	98%	74%	84%
(d) quality of client/patient care	90%	90%	85%	94%	94%	97%	90%	92%	74%	85%	78%	84%	97%	74%	68%	80%	94%
(c) access to clients'/patients' records	72%	78%	52%	77%	67%	99%	82%	71%	80%	89%	77%	81%	86%	88%	66%	86%	88%
(e) continuity of client/patient care	81%	82%	71%	85%	86%	94%	73%	84%	64%	76%	68%	84%	85%	69%	71%	62%	78%
(g) opportunity to get to know clients'/patients' families	64%	72%	49%	59%	64%	42%	65%	81%	64%	44%	50%	24%	8%	77%	50%	58%	28%
Number of nurses (= 100%)	824	457	171	132	64	291	371	102	1057	67	442	42	221	136	44	50	52

*Detailed answers to each of the six questions are given in the appendix at the end of the chapter.
†Q32 How would you assess the following things in your current work? Answers chosen from a card giving the ratings: very good, good, fair, poor, very poor.

4.6 Relationship between attitudes to clients/patients and attachment

Comparisons were made for district nurses, midwives and health visitors of the assessments of five of these six aspects of client/patient care made by nurses in different attachment/patch working situations. The sixth aspect— access to clients'/patients' records—is discussed in Chapter 5 along with the questions related to contact and relationships with GPs.

No differences between nurses with different attachment/patch working relationships were found on any of the five patient related issues for any of the three types of staff. Neither were there differences between nurses who worked with different numbers of practices. This suggests that these working arrangements bear no relation to nurses' assessment of these patient related aspects of their work.

Appendix to Chapter 4

Table A4.1 Assessment of the opportunity to get to know clients/patients, by type of nurse

Assessment	All DNs	DN SRN+	DN SRN –	DN SEN+	DN SEN –	GP empl.	Mid-wives	DN/ Midw.	HV	HV ass.	Schl. Nurse	Sch.N ass.	Fam. Plan.	Comm. Psych.	Geria-tric	Liai-son	Clinic
	%	%	%	%	%	%	%	%	%	%	%	%	%	%	%	%	%
Very good	49	52	40	49	50	54	43	50	39	36	26	26	23	60	50	46	46
Good	40	40	42	37	36	33	38	38	48	43	50	48	51	32	48	28	38
Fair	8	6	11	10	12	9	15	10	11	16	17	21	19	8	2	16	14
Poor	2	1	5	3	2	2	3	2	1	3	4	—	3	—	—	2	—
Very poor	1	*	1	1	—	—	—	—	*	—	1	—	1	—	—	2	—
Don't know/Did not answer/None	*	1	1	—	—	2	*	—	1	2	2	5	3	—	—	6	2
Number of nurses (= 100%)	824	457	171	132	64	291	371	102	1057	67	442	42	221	136	44	50	52

Table A4.2 Assessment of access to clients'/patients' records, by type of nurse

Assessment	All DNs	DN SRN+	DN SRN –	DN SEN+	DN SEN –	GP empl.	Mid-wives	DN/ Midw.	HV	HV ass.	Schl. Nurse	Sch.N ass.	Fam. Plan.	Comm. Psych.	Geria-tric	Liai-son	Clinic
	%	%	%	%	%	%	%	%	%	%	%	%	%	%	%	%	%
Very good	42	49	24	50	27	88	46	44	46	36	34	31	56	59	39	48	48
Good	30	29	28	27	40	11	36	27	34	53	43	50	30	29	27	38	40
Fair	11	9	13	11	15	1	11	15	10	6	9	3	3	9	11	4	6
Poor	8	7	12	7	8	—	4	6	4	—	5	3	3	3	7	4	2
Very poor	5	4	13	2	2	—	1	1	3	3	3	3	1	—	5	—	4
Don't know/Did not answer/None	4	2	10	3	8	*	2	7	3	2	6	10	7	—	11	6	—
Number of nurses (= 100%)	824	457	171	132	64	291	371	102	1057	67	442	42	221	136	44	50	52

Table A4.3 Assessment of quality of client/patient care, by type of nurse

Assessment	All DNs	DN SRN+	DN SRN –	DN SEN+	DN SEN –	GP empl.	Mid-Wives	DN/ Midw.	HV	HV ass.	Schl. Nurse	Sch.N ass.	Fam. Plan.	Comm. Psych.	Geria-tric	Liai-son	Clinic
	%	%	%	%	%	%	%	%	%	%	%	%	%	%	%	%	%
Very good	40	39	33	46	51	64	37	41	16	25	22	24	52	16	36	18	38
Good	50	51	52	48	43	33	53	51	58	60	56	60	45	58	32	62	56
Fair	9	9	14	6	6	3	9	7	23	12	15	5	3	21	30	14	—
Poor	*	*	*	—	—	*	1	—	1	—	1	—	*	2	2	—	2
Very poor	*	*	*	—	—	—	*	—	—	—	1	—	—	1	—	—	—
Don't know/Did not answer/None	1	1	1	—	—	*	—	1	2	3	5	11	—	2	—	4	4
Number of nurses (= 100%)	824	457	171	132	64	291	371	102	1057	67	442	42	221	136	44	50	52

Table A4.4 Assessment of continuity of client/patient care, by type of nurse

Assessment	All DNs	DN SRN+	DN SRN –	DN SEN+	DN SEN –	GP empl.	Mid-wives	DN/ Midw.	HV	HV ass.	Schl. Nurse	Sch.N ass.	Fam. Plan.	Comm. Psych.	Geria-tric	Liai-son	Clinic
	%	%	%	%	%	%	%	%	%	%	%	%	%	%	%	%	%
Very good	31	29	25	38	43	56	30	27	12	22	15	26	35	17	27	18	44
Good	50	53	46	47	43	38	43	57	52	54	53	58	50	52	44	44	34
Fair	15	15	23	10	12	5	21	13	29	16	24	5	10	23	27	30	10
Poor	3	2	4	4	2	*	4	1	5	5	3	—	1	6	2	—	2
Very poor	*	*	1	1	—	—	2	1	*	—	*	3	1	2	—	—	—
Don't know/Did not answer/None	1	1	1	—	*	1	*	1	2	3	5	8	3	—	—	8	10
Number of nurses (= 100%)	824	457	171	132	64	291	371	102	1057	67	442	42	221	136	44	50	52

Table A4.5 Assessment of knowledge of the geographical area worked in, by type of nurse

Assessment	All DNs	DN SRN+	DN SRN –	DN SEN+	DN SEN –	GP empl.	Mid-wives	DN/ Midw.	HV	HV ass.	Schl. Nurse	Sch.N ass.	Fam. Plan.	Comm. Psych.	Geria-tric	Liai-son	Clinic
	%	%	%	%	%	%	%	%	%	%	%	%	%	%	%	%	%
Very good	60	66	41	68	51	35	61	63	54	46	48	66	25	50	61	53	21
Good	33	30	40	30	35	23	32	25	37	39	40	24	29	34	34	39	29
Fair	7	4	17	2	12	12	6	11	8	9	8	5	10	12	5	8	4
Poor	*	—	1	—	2	3	1	1	1	4	2	3	4	3	—	—	13
Very poor	*	—	1	—	—	1	—	—	*	—	1	2	1	1	—	—	—
Don't know/Did not answer/None	*	*	*	—	—	26	—	—	*	2	1	—	31	—	—	—	33
Number of nurses (= 100%)	824	457	171	132	64	291	371	102	1057	67	442	42	221	136	44	50	52

Table A4.6 Assessment of opportunity to get to know clients'/patients' families, by type of nurse

Assessment	All DNs	DN SRN+	DN SRN −	DN SEN+	DN SEN −	GP empl.	Mid-wives	DN/ Midw.	HV	HV ass.	Schl. Nurse	Sch.N ass.	Fam. Plan.	Comm. Psych.	Geria-tric	Liai-son	Clinic
	%	%	%	%	%	%	%	%	%	%	%	%	%	%	%	%	%
Very good	26	30	20	23	24	18	24	35	20	10	15	3	1	31	14	10	17
Good	38	42	29	36	40	24	41	46	44	34	35	21	7	46	36	48	11
Fair	30	26	36	36	33	31	25	17	29	37	35	24	13	20	39	30	17
Poor	4	2	11	4	3	12	8	2	5	3	9	8	19	2	9	6	11
Very poor	1	*	2	1	—	3	1	—	1	8	2	10	13	—	2	—	6
Don't know/ Did not answer/ None	1	*	2	—	—	12	1	—	1	8	4	34	47	1	—	6	38
Number of nurses (= 100%)	824	457	171	132	64	291	371	102	1057	67	442	42	221	136	44	50	52

5 Contact and relationships with other primary health care staff

This chapter looks at nurses' views on relationships with other primary health care staff, particularly GPs. It also considers the effect of attachment and number of practices worked with on these relationships. It ends by examining the relative influence of attachment and number of practices worked with on nurses' attitudes towards general practice.

5.1 Membership of primary health care team
All nurses except auxiliaries were asked, 'Thinking about the way you work at the moment would you say you are a member of a primary health care team or not?' Table 5.1 shows the answers. As can be seen the large majority of all types of nurses regarded themselves as part of such a team. The one exception to this was community psychiatric nurses, only 39% of whom said they were a member of a primary health care team. This relates to their work base and as Table 3.8 showed, 81% of these nurses were based in hospitals. There was a similar relationship for liaison nurses 44% of whom were based in hospitals and 69%, rather lower than the norm, regarded themselves as members of a primary health care team. Rather surprisingly almost one quarter of health visitors did not regard themselves as members of a primary health care team.

5.2 Frequency of contact with GPs
Those types of nurses who can be formally attached to (or employed by) GPs—district nurses, midwives, health visitors, auxiliaries and GP employed nurses—were asked about the frequency of their contacts with GPs.* Table 5.2 shows that three quarters of auxiliaries had contact with their patients' GPs less often than once a week. In contrast most joint duty staff and district nurses with district training were in touch with GPs on five or more days each week. District nurses without district training had rather less contact than this. About one third of midwives and health visitors were in personal contact with GPs this often. It therefore appears that it is the district nurse function which leads to almost daily contact between a GP and a nurse.

5.3 Views on contacts and liaison with other staff
Nurses' opinions about communication with staff involved in health care in the community were collected. They were asked to assess their contacts and liaison about individual clients/patients with doctors, other primary health care staff, other nurses of the same type as themselves, their supervisor and social services staff.† Possible ratings were: very good, good, fair, poor or very poor. Some of the nurses replied that they had no contacts with some other types of staff. The full answers to the five questions are given in the appendix to this chapter but a summary is shown in Table 5.3. This gives the

*Q10 On average on how many working days per week do you have contact, either in the form of personal discussions or over the telephone, with any of your clients'/patients' GPs?

† See footnote to Table 5.3 for Q31

Table 5.1 Membership of a primary health care team, by type of nurse

Regarded themselves member of primary health care team	All DNs	DN SRN+	DN SRN –	DN SEN+	DN SEN –	GP empl.	Mid-wives	DN/ Midw.	HV	HV ass.	Schl. Nurse	Sch.N ass.	Fam. Plan.	Comm. Psych.	Geria-tric	Liai-son	Clinic
	%	%	%	%	%	%	%	%	%	%	%	%	%	%	%	%	%
Yes	84	83	79	91	89	84	88	92	77	92	86	86	85	39	91	69	77
No	16	17	21	9	11	16	12	8	23	8	14	14	15	61	9	31	23
Number of nurses (= 100%)	824	457	171	132	64	291	371	102	1057	67	442	42	221	136	44	50	52

Table 5.2 Average number of days in contact with GP, by type of nurse

Average number of days per week	All DNs	DN SRN+	DN SRN –	DN SEN+	DN SEN –	Auxil-iaries	GP empl.	Mid-wives	DN/ Midw.	HV	HV ass.
	%	%	%	%	%	%	%	%	%	%	%
Less than one	13	8	30	11	23	76	2	9	—	11	59
One	4	2	7	8	10	8	2	13	1	16	18
Two	7	5	11	11	13	3	6	16	5	19	5
Three	8	8	9	8	6	4	7	19	10	15	11
Four	8	9	8	3	6	1	16	11	8	8	2
Five or more	60	68	35	59	42	8	67	32	76	31	5
Number of nurses (= 100%)†	732	427	129	117	59	437††	291	350	94	1039	56

†Base numbers are smaller than on previous tables because full-time relief nurses, night sitters and bath nurses were excluded.

††This base is smaller than on previous comparable tables because one fifth of the nurses were not asked the question because of confusion at the interview about its relevance.

proportions who assessed contacts as very good or good. Nurses who had no contacts with a particular type of staff were included in the bases of these percentages so that the table shows—of all nurses, the proportion who had very good or good contacts and liaison.

The question was posed five times with the staff in the order a-e that is doctors were asked about first. However in Table 5.3 the staff are ranked in the order in which the total (weighted) sample of nurses rated their contacts. As can be seen contacts with other nurses of the same type were more frequently regarded as very good or good than contacts with the other categories of staff. Next came contacts with the supervisor and other primary health care staff. Contacts with doctors were overall ranked fourth and those with social services staff the least good.

Not surprisingly most of the largest groups of nurses—district nurses, midwives, health visitors, and school nurses all followed the same pattern. However auxiliaries rated contacts and liaison with their supervisor and other primary health care staff as better than contacts with other auxiliaries. GP employed nurses gave the highest assessment to GPs and the small proportion who assessed their contacts with supervisors as very good or good reflects the large proportion who had no supervisor. Overall however the main point to note from Table 5.3 is the very high proportions of all types of nurses who regarded their contacts and liaison with other nurses and doctors as very good or good.

5.4 Views on opportunities for discussions and meetings
The next table, Table 5.4, summarises the answers to four rather more specific questions asking nurses to assess their opportunities for discussions and meetings. Again, on the table the questions are ranked according to the proportion of all nurses who assessed their opportunities as very good or good.

The previous table (5.3) showed that joint district nurses/midwives were unusual in that a very high proportion of them, 92%, regarded their contacts and liaison with doctors as good or very good. This high rating of their communications with doctors is supported by their answers to the next question as shown in the first and third rows of Table 5.4. Eighty-nine per cent assessed their opportunities to discuss patients with doctors as very good or good and 82% similarly rated their opportunities to get to know GPs and their methods of working. These proportions are higher than for all other types of nurses apart from GP employed nurses who again rated their relationships with their employers very highly. Table 5.4 also shows that only a minority of specialist, that is school, family planning and community psychiatric nurses felt that their opportunities to get to know GPs were good. The majority of them however rated their opportunites to discuss patients with doctors as good or very good. The doctors in question of course are likely to be the relevant specialists rather than GPs.

For all types of nurses apart from GP employed ones opportunities for meetings with nursing officers and other staff in the district were more likely to be rated good or very good than opportunities for meetings with other primary health care staff.

Table 5.3 Summary table showing proportions rating contacts and liaison with different types of staff as very good or good†, by type of nurse

Assessment of contacts and liaison about individual patients with:	All DNs	DN SRN+	DN SRN −	DN SEN+	DN SEN −	Auxil-iaries	GP empl.	Mid-wives	DN/ Midw.	HV	HV ass.	Schl. Nurse	Sch.N ass.	Fam. Plan.	Comm. Psych.	Geria-tric	Liai-son	Clinic
(c) nurses of the same type	94%	96%	90%	91%	96%	60%	59%	97%	95%	94%	87%	93%	86%	88%	86%	82%	74%	76%
(d) supervisor	84%	84%	76%	88%	91%	89%	33%	87%	88%	78%	85%	88%	100%	67%	78%	94%	90%	79%
(b) other primary health care staff	78%	83%	64%	81%	83%	81%	88%	87%	84%	79%	88%	82%	84%	66%	63%	82%	78%	86%
(a) doctors	80%	86%	62%	83%	77%	46%	96%	84%	92%	71%	73%	65%	31%	81%	69%	61%	78%	70%
(e) social services staff	36%	32%	40%	43%	44%	30%	44%	33%	47%	45%	62%	31%	17%	26%	58%	50%	58%	43%
Number of nurses (= 100%)	*824*	*457*	*171*	*132*	*64*	*609*	*291*	*371*	*102*	*1057*	*67*	*442*	*42*	*221*	*136*	*44*	*50*	*52*

†Q.31 On the whole, how would you assess your contacts and liaison about individual clients/patients with:-(a)–(e)? Answers chosen from a card giving the ratings: very good, good, fair, poor, very poor.

Table 5.4 Summary table showing proportions rating opportunities for discussions and meetings as very good or good,† by type of nurse

(a) Assessment of opportunities	All DNs	DN SRN+	DN SRN −	DN SEN+	DN SEN −	Auxil-iaries	GP empl.	Mid-wives	DN/ Midw.	HV	HV ass.	Schl. Nurse	Sch.N ass.	Fam. Plan.	Comm. Psych.	Geria-tric	Liai-son	Clinic
32h to discuss patients with doctors	72%	78%	53%	77%	66%	—	93%	77%	89%	74%	61%	56%	13%	79%	74%	64%	74%	69%
31g for general meetings with nursing officers and other staff in the district	65%	69%	54%	64%	61%	57%	24%	64%	66%	66%	58%	54%	62%	42%	33%	41%	70%	56%
32b to get to know GPs and their methods of working	64%	72%	43%	64%	56%	—	95%	69%	82%	58%	33%	15%	11%	12%	27%	48%	22%	42%
31f for general meetings with other primary health care staff	39%	38%	30%	52%	42%	41%	39%	36%	48%	42%	36%	31%	36%	25%	32%	34%	38%	38%
Number of nurses (= 100%)	*824*	*457*	*171*	*132*	*64*	*609*	*291*	*371*	*102*	*1057*	*67*	*442*	*42*	*221*	*136*	*44*	*50*	*52*

† Q31. How would you assess the opportunities for more general meetings with:- (f), (g)?

Q32. How would you assess the following things in your current work?
    Answers chosen from a card giving the ratings: very good, good, fair, poor, very poor.

5.5 Contact with GPs by attachment

The nurses were also asked about the amount of contact they had with GPs† and the number of GPs and number of practices they worked with. These are considered next.

Table 5.5 shows the proportions of nurses with different patterns of attachment and their average number of days contact with GPs. The relationship between the different patterns of attachment and the amount of contact with GPs varied considerably with the type of nurse.

District nurses
The pattern was very clear for district nurses with attached district nurses having much more contact with GPs than those who were not attached. Seventy-four per cent of attached district nurses had contact with GPs on four or more days per week, on average, compared with only 32% of district nurses who were not attached. Forty-four per cent of the not attached district nurses had less than one day's contact per week with GPs, on average. Amongst the attached district nurses those who worked in all parts of the GP area only tended to have more contact with GPs than the others.

---

†Question 10 On average, on how many working days per week do you have contact, either in the form of personal discussions or over the telephone, with any of your patients' GPs?

Table 5.5 Average numbers of days per week in contact with GPs, by type of attachment

Average number of days	Not attached	Attached				
		All parts	Specific parts	All + patch	Specific + patch	All attached
District nurses	%	%	%	%	%	%
Less than one	44	5	9	11	8	7
1 – 3	24	17	20	21	31	19
4 or more	32	78	71	68	61	74
Number of district nurses (= 100%)	*126*	*336*	*87*	*105*	*66*	*594*
Midwives	%	%		%	%	%
Less than one	44	5	(1)	6	9	6
1 – 3	24	48	(10)	47	54	50
4 or more	32	47	(7)	47	37	44
Number of midwives (= 100%)	*66*	*114*	*18†*	*97*	*54*	*283*
Health visitors	%	%	%	%	%	%
Less than one	35	7	9	12	12	9
1 – 3	52	49	48	52	55	50
4 or more	13	44	43	36	33	41
Number of health visitors (= 100%)	*120*	*380*	*282*	*120*	*132*	*914*
Auxiliaries	%	%	%	%	%	%
Less than one	83	70	74	75	70	72
1 – 3	14	19	20	11	13	18
4 or more	3	11	6	14	17	10
Number of auxiliaries (= 100%)	*162*	*227*	*62*	*38*	*26*	*353*

† Percentages have not been calculated for groups where the bases are small. Actual numbers are given in brackets.

Midwives
Attached midwives also had more contact with GPs than the not attached. Forty-four per cent of the latter group were in contact on average less than one day per week compared with only six per cent of attached midwives.

Health visitors
Attached health visitors had more contact with GPs than the not attached. Forty-one per cent of the attached had an average four days contact per week with GPs compared with 13% of the not attached.

Auxiliaries
There was no difference between attached and not attached auxiliaries in the amount of contact they had with GPs.

Table 5.6 relates the different patterns of attachment to the number of GPs nurses worked with. Apart from auxiliaries, not attached nurses tended to work with larger numbers of GPs than attached nurses.

Table 5.6 Number of GPs worked with, by type of attachment

Number of GPs worked with	Not attached	Attached				
		All parts	Specific parts	All + patch	Specific + patch	All attached
District nurses	%	%	%	%	%	%
0 – 3†	12	33	21	21	22	28
4 – 6	12	51	56	39	33	48
7 – 10	9	12	17	23	27	16
11 or more	67	4	6	17	18	8
Number of district nurses (= 100%)	*126*	*336*	*87*	*105*	*66*	*594*
Midwives	%	%		%	%	%
0 – 3†	12	5	(2)	18	22	13
4 – 6	8	48	(7)	29	26	37
7 – 10	20	28	(7)	27	19	26
11 or more	60	19	(2)	26	33	24
Number of midwives (= 100%)	*66*	*114*	*18††*	*97*	*54*	*283*
Health visitors	%	%	%	%	%	%
0 – 3†	18	57	25	48	29	42
4 – 6	13	37	57	28	44	43
7 – 10	20	4	16	17	16	11
11 or more	49	2	2	7	11	4
Number of health visitors (= 100%)	*120*	*380*	*282*	*120*	*132*	*914*
Auxiliaries	%	%	%	%	%	%
0 – 3†	51	25	17	23	13	23
4 – 6	13	51	57	45	29	50
7 – 10	15	18	22	16	51	20
11 or more	21	6	4	16	17	7
Number of auxiliaries (= 100%)	*162*	*227*	*62*	*38*	*26*	*353*

† 0 – 3 includes nurses who had no contact with GPs.
†† Percentages have not been calculated for groups where the bases are small. Actual numbers are given in brackets.

District nurses
Of the attached district nurses those who worked an additional patch generally worked with more GPs than

those who did not have a patch; 40% of those working all areas plus a patch and 45% of those working specific areas plus a patch worked with seven or more GPs, compared with 16% and 23% of those without a patch.

Midwives
There were no differences between midwives with different attachments patterns.

Health visitors
The different attachment patterns of health visitors were related to the number of GPs they worked with. The attached health visitors who worked in all parts of the GP area only, tended to work with smaller numbers of GPs than the other attached health visitors, with 94% working for six GPs or less.

Auxiliaries
As the next table will show, almost one half of not attached auxiliaries had no contacts with general practitioners. This makes comparison with attached nurses difficult. Within the attached group there were no particular differences but the numbers in three of the categories were very small.

Table 5.7 shows the proportions of nurses working with different numbers of practices by the different patterns of attachment. The number of practices worked with is clearly related to the number of GPs worked with and so similar differences are found but a clearer pattern emerges. The nurses who were not attached worked with large numbers of practices. About three fifths of not attached district nurses, midwives and health visitors worked with five or more practices compared with one fifth or less of the attached nurses. The differences are smaller for midwives as a larger proportion of attached midwives than other types of nurse worked with two or more practices.

Looking at the attached nurses and their different patterns on attachment, nurses working an additional geographical patch (both those working in all parts of the GP's area and those in specific parts) tended to work with more practices than those without a patch. This was particularly true of district nurses and health visitors— around 60% of attached district nurses without a patch worked with only one practice and only a small percentage with five or more compared with around 35% of attached district nurses with a patch who worked with only one practice and around 20% who worked with five or more.

Among auxiliaries, a high proportion (46%) of the not attached did not work with GPs at all and this was the main difference between them and the attached auxiliaries. Again the attached nurses working an additional patch tended to work with larger numbers of practices than the attached nurses who did not have an additional patch.

5.6 Relationships with general practice by attachment
This section concentrates on those questions discussed in Sections 5.3 and 5.4 which refer to GPs and considers the

Table 5.7 Number of practices worked with, by type of attachment

Number of practices	Not attached	Attached				
		All parts	Specific parts	All + patch	Specific + patch	All attached
District nurses	%	%	%	%	%	%
One	4	63	61	35	38	55
Two	5	23	21	25	26	23
Three or four	19	11	11	19	18	10
Five or more	63	3	6	21	18	12
No GP contact	9	–	1	–	–	*
Number of district nurses (= 100%)	126	336	87	105	66	594
Midwives	%	%		%	%	%
One	10	21	(4)	21	26	22
Two	7	32	(7)	34	17	30
Three or four	17	36	(5)	19	24	28
Five or more	61	11	(2)	26	33	20
No GP contact	5	–	(–)	–	–	–
Number of midwives (= 100%)	66	114	18†	97	54	283
Health visitors	%	%	%	%	%	%
One	5	70	78	48	48	66
Two	5	23	13	31	23	21
Three or four	17	6	6	12	13	8
Five or more	59	1	3	9	16	5
No GP contact	14	*	–	–	–	*
Number of health visitors (= 100%)	120	380	282	120	132	914
Auxiliaries	%	%	%	%	%	%
One	8	52	49	36	26	49
Two	8	24	28	19	26	24
Three or four	16	20	16	26	31	20
Five or more	22	4	7	19	17	7
No GP contact	46	–	–	–	–	–
Number of auxiliaries (= 100%)	162	227	62	38	26	353

† Percentages have not been calculated for groups where the bases are small. Actual numbers are given in brackets.

effect of different patterns of attachment. Table 5.8 shows the proportion of nurses with different patterns of attachment who assessed as very good or good these aspects of their relationship with GPs. Each of the four major types of nurses—district nurses, midwives, health visitors and auxiliaries—is described separately as the relationship between attachment and relationships with GPs varied for the different types of nurses. The joint duty district nurse/midwives have been excluded from the following analysis because there were too few of them (102) for comparisons to be made between different patterns of working categories.

District nurses
Attached district nurses rated all aspects of their relationships with GPs much more highly than district nurses who were not attached. The question with least variation was whether nurses regarded themselves as members of a primary health care team—87% of attached nurses did, compared with 73% of nurses who were not attached. The proportion of attached nurses assessing the other aspects as very good or good ranged from 73% to

87% compared with a range of 36% to 58% for the not attached nurses.

There was some variation between district nurses with different patterns of attachment in their relationships with GPs. The attached district nurses who worked in all parts of the GP's area gave the highest ratings for all aspects of GP relationships. There was a general tendency for attached district nurses who worked an additional geographical patch to rate their relationships with GPs rather lower than those who did not have a patch to cover. In the same way those who covered all parts of the GP's area tended to have higher ratings than those working in specific parts of catchment areas. However these differences were rarely statistically significant for individual questions, one exception being access to patients' records which was less often rated as good by district nurses who worked an additional patch than by those without a patch.

Table 5.8 Some aspects of relationships with GPs, by type of attachment

Proportion assessed as very good or good	Not attached	Attached				
		All parts	Specific parts	All + patch	Specific + patch	All attached
District nurses						
Contacts and liaison with doctors	58%	90%	85%	79%	86%	87%
Opportunity to get to know GPs	36%	77%	68%	70%	68%	73%
Opportunity to discuss patients with doctors	43%	86%	78%	75%	73%	81%
Access to patients' records	44%	85%	82%	72%	68%	80%
Proportion regarded themselves members of a primary health care team	73%	89%	87%	85%	81%	87%
Number of district nurses (= 100%)	*126*	*336*	*87*	*105*	*66*	*594*
Midwives						
Contacts and liaison with doctors	80%	82%	(18)	86%	83%	85%
Opportunity to get to know GPs	49%	73%	(17)	79%	64%	75%
Opportunity to discuss patients with doctors	67%	77%	(17)	86%	75%	81%
Access to patients' records	70%	86%	(16)	90%	73%	85%
Proportion regarded themselves members of a primary health care team	78%	90%	(16)	95%	87%	91%
Number of midwives (= 100%)	*66*	*114*	*18†*	*97*	*54*	*283*

Proportion assessed as very good or good	Not attached	Attached				
		All parts	Specific parts	All + patch	Specific + patch	All attached
Health visitors						
Contacts and liaison with doctors	47%	79%	68%	77%	68%	74%
Opportunity to get to know GPs	26%	69%	55%	63%	55%	62%
Opportunity to discuss patients with doctors	46%	81%	76%	77%	70%	77%
Access to patients' records	52%	86%	86%	77%	73%	83%
Proportion regarded themselves members of a primary health care team	48%	83%	83%	78%	73%	81%
Number of health visitors (= 100%)	*120*	*380*	*282*	*120*	*132*	*914*
Auxiliaries						
Contacts and liaison with doctors	33%	58%	44%	61%	67%	57%
Number of auxiliaries (= 100%)	*162*	*227*	*62*	*38*	*26*	*353*

† Percentages have not been calculated for these groups where the bases are small. Actual numbers are given in brackets.

Midwives

All midwives both attached and not attached, rated their contacts and liaisons with doctors highly and there was little variation between those working different types of attachment. There was more variation in the other aspects of their relationships with GPs with attached midwives rating them more highly, particularly the opportunity to get to know GPs which was assessed as very good or good by 75% of attached midwives compared with 49% of midwives who were not attached.

Considering the different patterns of attachment, those who worked in all parts of the GP's area and had an additional geographical patch consistently had the highest proportions of very good or good ratings, generally followed by those working all parts only. Those working specific areas plus a patch usually had the lowest proportions. Only 18 midwives worked specific parts of the GP's area, so this group was too small to consider.

Health visitors

The variation between attached and not attached health visitors was almost as marked as for district nurses, with all aspects of the relationships with GPs rated much lower by the not attached health visitors, even membership of the primary health care team. In particular the opportunity to get to know GPs, generally rated low by health visitors, was rated as very good or good by only 26% of health visitors who were not attached compared with 62% of attached health visitors.

Comparing the different patterns of attachment, whether the health visitor worked all parts or specific parts of the GP area seemed to be the important factor for the first two questions about GP relationships listed on the table. Those working all parts of the area (both with and without an additional patch) rated these two aspects more highly than those working in specific parts of the catchment area.

Auxiliaries
Auxiliaries were not asked most of the questions about relationships with GPs. The only question they were asked was to assess their contacts and liaison with doctors about individual patients. Again there was a difference between the attached and not attached staff, a higher proportion of the attached rated their contacts as very good or good.

5.7 Analysis by number of practices worked with
As the previous section showed, nurses with different attachment and patch working arrangements varied greatly in the number of general practices that they worked with. Generally speaking therefore, those who were not attached and those who worked an additional patch worked with a larger number of practices than those who were only attached to practices. It seemed reasonable to suppose that the number of practices nurses worked with would be related to aspects of their work and opinions in the same way as their attachment arrangements. The analyses carried out for the previous sections of this chapter were therefore repeated comparing nurses working with different numbers of practices.

The results were very similar to those found when nurses with different attachment patterns were compared. Again it is worth pointing out that there were no differences at all for any of the nurses in their assessments of the patient related aspects of their work. This section concentrates on some key questions relating to relationships with GPs.

Table 5.9 shows how the number of practices worked with was related to the average number of days per week that nurses were in contact† with GPs. As can be seen for all four types of nurse the larger the number of practices worked with the lower the number of days on which they had personal contact with their patients' doctors.

Table 5.10 shows the proportions of nurses who regarded themselves as members of a primary health care team and the proportions who assessed various other aspects of their relationship with general practice as good or very good. (See Q 32.)

District nurses
There was a clear trend for district nurses who worked with larger numbers of practices to be less likely to regard themselves as members of a primary health care team. Some 91% of district nurses working with only one practice regarded themselves part of one, this fell to

---

†Q10 On average on how many working days per week do you have contact, either in the form of personal discussions or over the telephone with any of your clients'/patients' GPs?

Table 5.9 Average number of days per week in contact with GPs, by number of practices worked with

Average number of days	Number of practices				
	One	Two	Three	Four	Five or more
District nurses	%	%	%	%	%
Less than one	5	5	8	16	40
1 – 3	16	22	31	24	24
4 or more	79	73	61	60	36
Number of district nurses (= 100%)	*327*	*142*	*65*	*34*	*117*
Midwives	%	%	%	%	%
Less than one	3	5	5	16	17
1 – 3	41	59	50	52	43
4 or more	56	36	45	32	40
Number of midwives (= 100%)	*68*	*88*	*62*	*25*	*92*
Health visitors	%	%	%	%	%
Less than one	7	9	23	15	30
1 – 3	48	54	52	65	49
4 or more	45	37	25	20	21
Number of health visitors (= 100%)	*610*	*196*	*56*	*34*	*111*
Auxiliaries	%	%	%	%	%
Less than one	65	77	74	80	83
1 – 3	22	15	18	12	14
4 or more	13	8	8	8	3
Number of auxiliaries (= 100%)	*173*	*90*	*65*	*40*	*53*

73% of district nurses who worked with five or more practices. There was a similar downward trend for access to patients' records. However for the first three questions shown in Table 5.11, assessing contacts and liaison with doctors, opportunity to get to know doctors and to discuss patients with doctors, the downward trend in the proportions assessing them as good or very good began only with district nurses working with three or four practices. Those working with one or two practices held similar views.

Midwives
The downward trends associated with number of practices worked with were much less marked for midwives than for district nurses and health visitors although the group who worked with five or more practices consistently gave less favourable assessments of these aspects of their relationship with GPs.

Health visitors
Health visitors were similar to district nurses in that there were downward trends for each of the five questions. Moreover for health visitors there were differences for each question between those who worked with one practice only and those who worked with two.

5.8 Attachment and number of practices worked with
The findings discussed in the previous section suggest that number of practices worked with was a powerful factor influencing community nurses' relationships with general practice. But it was also highly correlated with attachment and patch working arrangements. It is

therefore important to try to assess the relative importance of the two factors. To do this it is necessary to look at attached and not attached nurses separately to analyse number of practices worked with by relationships with and views on general practice.

Less than one fifth of nurses who could be attached to general practice were not attached in some way. Thus comparing attached and not attached nurses in the above way is only possible if the different types of nurses are considered together. Table 5.11 repeats the analysis in Table 5.10 considering attached and not attached nurses separately. The table includes district nurses, midwives, district nurse/midwives and health visitors. We have been unable to consider district nurse/midwives separately in this chapter because there were too few of them (102) but it is appropriate to include them in this analysis. Auxiliaries are excluded because few had direct contact with GPs and were not asked most of the questions considered.

As the previous section showed there are similar trends for each of the five attitude questions. For attached nurses there was a clear downward trend in the proportion of nurses expressing positive views towards general practice with the increase in number of practices worked with. In general the differences were between three groups—those who worked with one practice, two or three practices and four or more practices. However this was not true for one question—opportunities to get to know GPs. The differences between nurses who worked with one practice and those who worked with two or three were smaller than the differences between those who worked with two or three and those who worked with four or more practices.

For not attached nurses there was a more marked downward trend except that those working with one practice did not follow the general pattern. This may not be surprising since the 20 nurses working with one practice but not formally attached were likely to have been in unusual work situations.

Table 5.10 Some aspects of relationships with GPs, by number of practices worked with

Proportion assessed as very good or good	Number of practices				
	One	Two	Three	Four	Five or more
District nurses					
Contacts and liaison with doctors	89%	88%	88%	78%	61%
Opportunity to get to know GPs	78%	78%	76%	52%	36%
Opportunity to discuss patients with doctors	85%	84%	85%	63%	50%
Access to patients' records	88%	79%	74%	59%	45%
Proportion regarded themselves members of a primary health care team	91%	85%	82%	79%	73%
Number of district nurses (= 100%)	*327*	*142*	*65*	*34*	*117*
Midwives					
Contacts and liaison with doctors	90%	83%	84%	83%	81%
Opportunity to get to know GPs	72%	81%	78%	72%	58%
Opportunity to discuss patients with doctors	79%	89%	77%	79%	72%
Access to patients' records	88%	91%	89%	84%	64%
Proportion regarded themselves members of a primary health care team	93%	98%	82%	88%	84%
Number of midwives (= 100%)	*68*	*88*	*62*	*25*	*92*
Health visitors					
Contacts and liaison with doctors	78%	66%	64%	55%	53%
Opportunity to get to know GPs	65%	59%	54%	41%	37%
Opportunity to discuss patients with doctors	81%	73%	75%	64%	45%
Access to patients' records	90%	76%	66%	62%	44%
Proportion regarded themselves members of a primary health care team	86%	73%	70%	62%	52%
Number of health visitors (= 100%)	*610*	*196*	*56*	*34*	*111*

Table 5.11 Relationship between attachment, number of practices worked with and nurses' views on relationships with general practice

Views on relationships with general practice	Attachment and number of practices worked with											
	Attached						Not attached					
	1	2	3	4	5+	All	1	2	3	4	5+	All
Regarded themselves members of a primary health care team	89%	83%	80%	77%	79%	85%	90%	90%	77%	74%	63%	68%
Assessed as very good or good – contacts and liaison with doctors	84%	80%	81%	74%	76%	82%	80%	90%	80%	70%	54%	62%
Assessed as very good or good – opportunities to get to know GPs	72%	72%	72%	56%	55%	70%	55%	90%	70%	51%	30%	41%
Assessed as very good or good – opportunities to discuss patients with doctors	83%	81%	80%	66%	69%	80%	65%	85%	77%	67%	42%	52%
Assessed as very good or good – access to patients' records	88%	78%	75%	67%	61%	82%	80%	75%	83%	60%	40%	50%
Number of district nurses, midwives, district nurse/midwives and health visitors (= 100%)	*1361*	*563*	*225*	*89*	*206*	*2444*	*20*	*20*	*30*	*43*	*244*	*357*

Table 5.12 summarises Table 5.11. The number of practices worked with has been grouped into two categories—one to three and four or more. From part a) of Table 5.12 it can be seen that on each of the five questions the number of practices worked with was a significant factor when attached and not attached nurses were considered separately. For example access to patients' records was regarded as good or very good by 84% of attached nurses working with one to three practices but by only 63% of attached nurses working with four or more practices. There was an even greater difference between the two groups of not attached nurses—80% compared with 43%.

Part b) of Table 5.12 is a re-arrangement of part a) showing the differences between attached and not attached nurses when number of practices worked with is held constant. The table shows no difference between attached and not attached nurses who worked with a small number of practices but large differences between those who worked with four or more practices. Thus there is no simple answer to the question of which of the two factors—attachment or number of practices worked with—is most important in relation to nurses' views on general practice. However the number of practices worked with appears to have a greater effect than attachment.

Separate analysis of attached district nurses, midwives and health visitors by the number of practices they worked with was possible. This confirmed for each of these three groups of nurses the downward trends in proportions having positive views of general practice as the number of practices they worked with increased. The trends were less marked among the smallest group—midwives—than they were for the two largest groups of nurses working in the community—district nurses and health visitors.

Table 5.12 Summary table showing the relationship between attachment, number of practices worked with and nurses' views on relationships with general practice

Views on relationships with general practice	(a) Attachment and number of practices worked with						(b) Number of practices worked with and attachment					
	Attached			Not attached			1 – 3			4 or more		
	1–3	4+	Stat. sig. diff. †	1–3	4+	Stat. sig. diff. †	Atta-ched	Not att.	Stat. sig. diff. †	Atta-ched	Not att.	Stat. sig. diff.†
Regarded themselves members of a primary health care team	86%	78%	√	84%	64%	√	86%	84%	×	78%	64%	√
Assessed as very good or good-contacts and liaison with doctors	82%	76%	√	83%	56%	√	82%	83%	×	76%	33%	√
Assessed as very good or good – opportunities to get to know GPs	72%	56%	√	71%	33%	√	72%	71%	×	56%	33%	√
Assessed as very good or good – opportunities to discuss patients with doctors	82%	68%	√	76%	46%	√	82%	76%	×	68%	46%	√
Assessed as very good or good – access to patients' records	84%	63%	√	80%	43%	√	84%	80%	×	63%	43%	√
Number of district nurses, midwives, district nurse/midwives and health visitors (= 100%)	2149	295		70	287		2149	70		295	287	

† √ denotes a difference which is statistically significant at the 95% level.
  × denotes a difference which is not statistically significant at the 95% level.

Appendix to Chapter 5

Table A5.1 Assessment of contacts and liaison with doctors about individual clients/patients, by type of nurse

Assessment	All DNs	DN SRN+	DN SRN−	DN SEN+	DN SEN−	Auxil-iaries	GP empl.	Mid-wives	DN/ Midw.	HV	HV ass.	Schl. Nurse	Sch.N ass.	Fam. Plan.	Comm. Psych.	Geria-tric	Liai-son	Clinic
	%	%	%	%	%	%	%	%	%	%	%	%	%	%	%	%	%	%
Very good	47	54	34	48	32	25	74	50	61	32	31	28	12	51	31	36	32	47
Good	33	32	28	35	45	21	22	34	31	39	42	37	19	30	38	25	46	23
Fair	12	9	21	10	15	7	3	14	7	22	10	16	7	10	24	23	10	12
Poor	3	3	6	4	1	4	−	1	−	5	5	7	−	3	4	14	4	−
Very poor	2	1	3	2	−	2	−	*	1	1	−	2	−	1	1	−	−	2
Don't know/ Did not answer/ None	3	1	8	1	7	41	1	1	−	1	12	10	62	5	2	2	8	16
Number of nurses (= 100%)	824	457	171	132	64	609	291	371	102	1057	67	442	42	221	136	44	50	52

Table A5.2 Assessment of contacts and liaison with other primary health care staff about individual clients/patients, by type of nurse

Assessment	All DNs	DN SRN+	DN SRN−	DN SEN+	DN SEN−	Auxil-iaries	GP empl.	Mid-wives	DN/ Midw.	HV	HV ass.	Schl. Nurse	Sch.N ass.	Fam. Plan.	Comm. Psych.	Geria-tric	Liai-son	Clinic
	%	%	%	%	%	%	%	%	%	%	%	%	%	%	%	%	%	%
Very good	39	41	28	47	41	53	56	48	47	34	45	37	43	28	20	36	28	59
Good	39	42	36	34	42	28	32	39	37	45	43	45	41	38	43	46	50	27
Fair	15	12	24	15	11	7	9	9	15	17	8	13	7	12	29	11	10	8
Poor	4	3	9	3	3	2	*	2	−	3	1	2	2	4	4	5	6	−
Very poor	1	1	−	1	−	2	−	*	−	*	−	−	−	1	2	2	−	2
Don't know/ Did not answer/ None	2	1	3	−	3	8	3	2	1	1	3	3	7	17	2	−	6	4
Number of nurses (= 100%)	824	457	171	132	64	609	291	371	102	1057	67	442	42	221	136	44	50	52

Table A5.3 Assessment of contacts and liaison with other nurses of the same type about individual clients/patients, by type of nurse

Assessment	All DNs	DN SRN+	DN SRN−	DN SEN+	DN SEN−	Auxil-iaries	GP empl.	Mid-wives	DN/ Midw.	HV	HV ass.	Schl. Nurse	Sch.N ass.	Fam. Plan.	Comm. Psych.	Geria-tric	Liai-son	Clinic
	%	%	%	%	%	%	%	%	%	%	%	%	%	%	%	%	%	%
Very good	59	62	53	56	68	38	44	71	68	51	54	59	53	54	49	41	44	52
Good	35	34	37	35	28	22	15	26	27	43	33	34	33	34	37	41	30	24
Fair	4	3	7	4	3	3	1	2	5	4	1	3	2	2	5	−	8	4
Poor	1	*	1	2	−	2	1	−	−	*	1	1	2	1	3	7	2	−
Very poor	*	−	*	−	−	1	1	*	−	*	−	−	−	*	1	−	−	2
Don't know/ Did not answer/ None	1	1	2	3	1	34	38	1	−	2	11	3	10	9	5	11	16	18
Number of nurses (= 100%)	824	457	171	132	64	609	291	371	102	1057	67	442	42	221	136	44	50	52

Table A5.4 Assessment of contacts and liaison with supervisor about individual clients/patients, by type of nurse

Assessment	All DNs	DN SRN+	DN SRN−	DN SEN+	DN SEN−	Auxil-iaries	GP empl.	Mid-wives	DN/ Midw.	HV	HV ass.	Schl. Nurse	Sch.N ass.	Fam. Plan.	Comm. Psych.	Geria-tric	Liai-son	Clinic
	%	%	%	%	%	%	%	%	%	%	%	%	%	%	%	%	%	%
Very good	48	44	40	59	65	66	29	55	44	36	57	44	50	37	43	64	58	57
Good	36	40	36	29	26	23	4	32	44	42	28	44	50	30	35	30	32	22
Fair	10	9	14	9	8	5	1	8	6	14	6	9	−	11	7	4	2	4
Poor	2	2	3	1	1	1	*	2	3	2	2	1	−	5	5	2	−	−
Very poor	1	1	3	−	−	1	*	1	2	1	−	*	−	2	4	*	−	4
Don't know/ Did not answer/ None	3	4	4	2	−	4	66	2	1	5	7	2	−	15	6	−	8	13
Number of nurses (= 100%)	824	457	171	132	64	609	291	371	102	1057	67	442	42	221	136	44	50	52

Table A5.5 Assessment of contacts and liaison with social services staff about individual clients/patients, by type of nurse

Assessment	All DNs	DN SRN+	DN SRN−	DN SEN+	DN SEN−	Auxil-iaries	GP empl.	Mid-wives	DN/ Midw.	HV	HV ass.	Schl. Nurse	Sch.N ass.	Fam. Plan.	Comm. Psych.	Geria-tric	Liai-son	Clinic
	%	%	%	%	%	%	%	%	%	%	%	%	%	%	%	%	%	%
Very good	9	8	10	11	12	13	20	10	12	10	18	7	7	8	20	11	24	18
Good	27	24	30	32	32	17	24	23	35	35	44	24	10	18	38	39	34	25
Fair	35	41	22	28	36	8	12	27	30	39	22	27	9	18	26	39	26	2
Poor	13	15	12	13	6	5	7	9	12	12	3	13	5	6	10	−	4	−
Very poor	7	7	5	9	−	3	4	4	8	3	−	5	5	4	4	4	8	−
Don't know/ Did not answer/ None	9	5	21	7	14	54	33	27	3	1	13	24	64	46	2	7	4	55
Number of nurses (= 100%)	824	457	171	132	64	609	291	371	102	1057	67	442	42	221	136	44	50	52

Table A5.6 Assessment of the opportunities for general meetings with other primary health care staff, by type of nurse

Assessment	All DNs	DN SRN+	DN SRN-	DN SEN+	DN SEN-	Auxil-iaries	GP empl.	Mid-wives	DN/ Midw.	HV	HV ass.	Schl. Nurse	Sch. N ass.	Fam. Plan.	Comm. Psych.	Geria-tric	Liai-son	Clinic
	%	%	%	%	%	%	%	%	%	%	%	%	%	%	%	%	%	%
Very good	10	10	9	13	12	11	14	11	9	10	2	6	12	6	7	4	8	10
Good	29	28	21	39	30	30	25	25	39	32	34	25	24	19	25	30	30	28
Fair	31	33	29	28	29	14	17	31	22	32	33	33	12	20	36	23	34	14
Poor	15	16	16	11	8	13	11	16	15	17	10	17	10	20	23	30	18	14
Very poor	5	4	8	4	9	4	7	6	4	3		4	2	8	5	9	2	2
Don't know/Did not answer/ None	10	9	17	5	12	28	26	11	11	6	21	15	40	27	4	4	8	32
Number of nurses (= 100%)	*824*	*457*	*171*	*132*	*64*	*609*	*291*	*371*	*102*	*1057*	*67*	*442*	*42*	*221*	*136*	*44*	*50*	*52*

Table A5.7 Assessment of opportunities for general meetings with nursing officers and other staff in the district, by type of nurse

Assessment	All DNs	DN SRN+	DN SRN-	DN SEN+	DN SEN-	Auxil-iaries	GP empl.	Mid-wives	DN/ Midw.	HV	HV ass.	Schl. Nurse	Sch. N ass.	Fam. Plan.	Comm. Psych.	Geria-tric	Liai-son	Clinic
	%	%	%	%	%	%	%	%	%	%	%	%	%	%	%	%	%	%
Very good	17	16	13	21	25	19	6	20	7	13	7	11	14	7	9	-	24	21
Good	48	53	41	43	36	38	18	44	59	53	51	43	48	35	24	41	46	35
Fair	21	20	25	24	22	13	7	23	24	22	19	26	5	19	32	23	12	18
Poor	6	5	9	7	8	7	13	5	6	6	-	9	5	18	18	21	16	6
Very poor	2	2	2	1	1	3	7	2	2	1	2	3	2	4	5	11	2	6
Don't know/Did not answer/ None	6	4	10	4	8	20	49	6	2	5	21	8	26	17	12	4	-	14
Number of nurses (= 100%)	*824*	*457*	*171*	*132*	*64*	*609*	*291*	*371*	*102*	*1057*	*67*	*442*	*42*	*221*	*136*	*44*	*50*	*52*

Table A5.8 Assessment of the opportunity to get to know GPs and their methods of working, by type of nurse

Assessment	All DNs	DN SRN+	DN SRN-	DN SEN+	DN SEN-	GP empl.	Mid-wives	DN/ Midw.	HV	HV ass.	Schl. Nurse	Sch. N ass.	Fam. Plan.	Comm. Psych.	Geria-tric	Liai-son	Clinic
	%	%	%	%	%	%	%	%	%	%	%	%	%	%	%	%	%
Very good	30	38	13	27	22	70	33	46	22	5	4	3	6	6	23	4	21
Good	34	34	30	37	34	25	36	36	36	28	11	8	6	21	25	18	21
Fair	21	17	28	27	22	5	23	15	28	36	27	3	17	35	25	28	17
Poor	9	7	17	6	11	*	5	3	10	12	26	8	28	29	20	24	14
Very poor	3	2	5	2	2	-	1	-	2	3	11	3	10	6	7	2	4
Don't know/Did not answer/ None	3	2	7	1	9	*	2	-	2	16	21	75	33	3	-	24	23
Number of nurses (= 100%)	*824*	*457*	*171*	*132*	*64*	*291*	*371*	*102*	*1057*	*67*	*442*	*42*	*221*	*136*	*44*	*50*	*52*

Table A5.9 Assessment of the opportunity to discuss clients/patients with doctors, by type of nurse

Assessment	All DNs	DN SRN+	DN SRN-	DN SEN+	DN SEN-	GP empl.	Mid-wives	DN/ Midw.	HV	HV ass.	Schl. Nurse	Sch.N ass.	Fam. Plan.	Comm. Psych.	Geria-tric	Liai-son	Clinic
	%	%	%	%	%	%	%	%	%	%	%	%	%	%	%	%	%
Very good	41	49	23	37	39	68	37	61	33	18	20	5	47	39	25	33	48
Good	31	29	30	40	27	25	40	28	41	43	36	8	32	35	39	41	21
Fair	15	14	19	14	19	5	18	10	19	21	19	8	7	21	14	24	6
Poor	6	4	12	7	3	1	4	1	5	3	12	3	5	4	16	2	4
Very poor	3	2	7	2	2	*	*	-	1	2	3	5	2	1	-	-	4
Don't know/Did not answer/ None	4	2	9	-	10	1	1	-	1	13	10	71	7	-	6	-	17
Number of nurses (= 100%)	*824*	*457*	*171*	*132*	*64*	*291*	*371*	*102*	*1057*	*67*	*442*	*42*	*221*	*136*	*44*	*50*	*52*

6 Travelling and time spent at different locations

An important feature of working in the community is the need for nurses to travel in order to visit patients, clients, clinics and stores. This chapter describes the nurses' method of travel and their views on travelling and then goes on to examine information from the diaries about the amount of time actually spent on travelling by the different types of nurses working in the community.

6.1 Method of travel and views on travel

All the nurses were asked 'When you make visits either to clients/patients or other places as part of your work, how do you normally travel?' Only among GP practice nurses, family planning and clinic nurses did substantial proportions of staff not make visits. These are shown in Table 6.1 together with the method of travel used. Virtually all the nurses who travelled as part of their work did so by car. However about one tenth of auxiliaries, school, geriatric and clinic nurses used public transport. In addition just over one tenth of the latter two groups and of health visitor and school nurse assistants walked. Hardly any nurses used two wheeled methods of transport.

The nurses were also asked about their views on the amount of travelling they did†. Their answers are given in Table 6.2. Rather surprisingly perhaps most nurses felt that the amount of travelling they did was 'about right'. However about one third of midwives, district nurse/midwives, community psychiatric and geriatric nurses felt that they did too much or far too much travelling. This was also true for one quarter of district nurses and health visitors.

†Q16 How do you feel about the amount of travelling involved in your job? Is it far too much, too much or is it about right?

6.2 Attachment and number of practices worked with and views on travel

Table 6.3 investigates differences in the views of attached and not attached nurses on the amount of travelling they did. Within the attached group, variations between those with different attachment and patch working patterns are also shown. For each of the four main types of nurses† (district nurses, midwives, health visitors and auxiliaries) the table shows the proportions of nurses who used a car for visits and the proportions who regarded the amount of travelling they did as too much or far too much.

Virtually all *district nurses* used a car for visits and there were no differences between any of the attachment categories. Neither was there a difference between the not attached and the total group of attached district nurses in the proportions who regarded the amount of travel as excessive. However those attached nurses who worked a patch in addition to all or part of a GP area were more likely than nurses without a patch to regard the amount of travel as too much.

Nearly all *midwives* used a car for visits and there were no differences between those in different attachment categories. Having an additional patch was not related to the proportion of attached midwives regarding the amount of travel as excessive. However a higher proportion of all attached midwives than of not attached midwives regarded the amount of travel they did as too or far too much, 34% compared with 23%.

†Full-time relief nurses in all groups have been excluded as have bath attendants and night sitters from the auxiliaries group. These nurses were not asked the questions about attachment to general practice.

Table 6.1 Method of travel for visits, by type of nurse

Method of travel	All DNs	DN SRN+	DN SRN–	DN SEN+	DN SEN–	Auxil-iaries	GP empl.	Mid-wives	DN/ Midw.	HV	HV ass.	Schl. Nurse	Sch.N ass.	Fam. Plan.	Comm. Psych.	Geria-tric	Liai-son	Clinic
	%	%	%	%	%	%	%	%	%	%	%	%	%	%	%	%	%	%
Car	99	99	98	99	98	81	30	98	100	93	82	81	60	49	98	82	90	25
Public transport	*	–	–	–	–	11	1	1	–	2	3	8	24	4	1	7	–	10
On foot	*	*	–	–	–	4	2	*	–	4	12	7	10	1	–	11	6	13
Bicycle	1	1	*	1	–	*	1	1	–	1	–	1	2	1	1	–	–	–
Motorbike/moped/other	–	–	1	–	2	1	1	–	–	–	1	2	2	*	–	2	–
Does not make visits	*	*	1	–	–	3	65	*	–	–	2	1	2	45	–	–	2	52
Number of nurses (= 100%)	*824*	*457*	*171*	*132*	*64*	*609*	*291*	*371*	*102*	*1057*	*67*	*442*	*42*	*221*	*136*	*44*	*50*	*52*

Table 6.2 Views on amount of travelling, by type of nurse

Views on travel	All DNs	DN SRN+	DN SRN–	DN SEN+	DN SEN–	Auxil-iaries	GP empl.	Mid-wives	DN/ Midw.	HV	HV ass.	Schl. Nurse	Sch.N ass.	Fam. Plan.	Comm. Psych.	Geria-tric	Liai-son	Clinic
	%	%	%	%	%	%	%	%	%	%	%	%	%	%	%	%	%	%
Far too much	6	5	6	9	2	2	–	11	12	6	1	2	–	2	7	7	6	–
Too much	17	17	19	20	10	7	2	22	24	19	3	5	–	7	31	23	2	–
About right	77	78	74	71	88	88	31	67	64	64	75	94	91	95	46	62	70	86	46
Too little (spontaneous answer)	–	–	–	–	–	*	2	*	–	*	–	1	3	–	–	–	4	2
Does not make visits	*	*	1	–	–	3	65	*	–	–	2	1	2	45	–	–	2	52
Number of nurses (= 100%)	*824*	*457*	*171*	*132*	*64*	*609*	*291*	*371*	*102*	*1057*	*67*	*442*	*42*	*221*	*136*	*44*	*50*	*52*

Table 6.3 Method of transport and views on amount of travel, by type of attachment

	Not attached	Attached				
		All parts	Specific parts	All + patch	Specific + patch	All attached
District nurses						
Proportion using car for visits	97%	99%	97%	97%	100%	99%
Proportion regarding amount of travel as too much or far too much	20%	22%	18%	26%	28%	23%
Number of district nurses† *(= 100%)*	*126*	*336*	*87*	*105*	*66*	*594*
Midwives						
Proportion using car for visits	93%	99%	(17)	98%	98%	99%
Proportion regarding amount of travel as too much or far too much	23%	37%	(4)	34%	32%	34%
Number of midwives† *(= 100%)*	*66*	*114*	*18††*	*97*	*54*	*283*
Health visitors						
Proportion using car for visits	80%	97%	93%	97%	91%	95%
Proportion regarding amount of travel as too much or far too much	19%	30%	22%	26%	23%	26%
Number of health visitors† *(= 100%)*	*120*	*380*	*282*	*120*	*132*	*914*
Auxiliaries						
Proportion using car for visits	68%	95%	83%	91%	92%	93%
Proportion regarding amount of travel as too much or far too much	9%	5%	9%	11%	17%	7%
Number of auxiliaries† *(= 100%)*	*162*	*227*	*62*	*38*	*26*	*353*

†Full-time relief nurses, bath attendants and night sitters were not asked about attachment and so are not included in the table.
††Percentages have not been calculated for groups where the bases are small. Actual numbers are given in brackets.

Table 6.4 Method of transport and views on amount of travel, by number of practices worked with

	Number of practices			
	1	2	3–4	5+
District nurses				
Proportion using car for visits	99%	98%	98%	98%
Proportion regarding amoung of travel as too much or far too much	18%	24%	34%	23%
Number of district nurses *(= 100%)*	*327*	*142*	*98*	*117*
Midwives				
Proportion using car for visits	99%	98%	98%	97%
Proportion regarding amount of travel as too much or far too much	34%	30%	32%	34%
Number of midwives *(= 100%)*	*68*	*88*	*87*	*92*
Health visitors				
Proportion using car for visits	94%	98%	97%	81%
Proportion regarding amount of travel as too much or far too much	23%	30%	37%	21%
Number of health visitors *(= 100%)*	*610*	*196*	*90*	*111*
Auxiliaries				
Proportion using car for visits	92%	92%	86%	85%
Proportion regarding amount of travel as too much or far too much	7%	6%	7%	13%
Number of auxiliaries *(= 100%)*	*173*	*90*	*90*	*53*

More attached *health visitors* than the not attached used a car for visits, 95% compared with 80%. Also 97% of those covering all parts of a GP area used a car compared with 92% of those attached health visitors who covered only part of a GP area. The same pattern of differences can be observed in Table 6.3 in the proportions who regarded the amount of travel as too much; excessive travelling was reported more commonly by the attached than the not attached and by those covering all parts of a catchment area than by those covering just specific parts.

Attached *auxiliaries* were more likely than the not attached to use cars for their visits, 93% did compared with 68%. However there were no differences between attached nurses with different working arrangements. A similar proportion of auxiliaries in each of the attachment categories reported the amount of travel they did as excessive.

In summary then, attached health visitors and auxiliaries more often used cars for visits than the not attached. There was some indication that for district nurses, midwives and health visitors attachment itself or the working of additional patches or covering the whole of a GP area resulted in perceived excessive travel. However these difference although statistically significant were not large.

Table 6.4 looks at the variation in car use and views on travel between nurses working with different numbers of practices. There were no differences in car use between district nurses, midwives and auxiliaries, but amongst health visitors those working with five or more practices were less likely to use a car. There were no significant differences for midwives and auxiliaries in the proportion who regarded the amount of travel as too much or far too much. For district nurses and health visitors those working with three or four practices had the highest proportions who regarded their travel as too much or far too much.

We now use information from the diaries to look at the actual time spent travelling by the different types of nurses. First, then, we must introduce the diary and explain how it was completed and what information was collected.

6.3 Description of the diary information
Detailed information about the work carried out by the different kinds of nurses working in the community was obtained from diaries completed by the nurses. Each nurse completed a diary recording all work activities (including travel) for seven days, beginning the day after the day they were interviewed. For most nurses the seven days included two non-working days at weekends. Days off sick or on leave were recorded as such. For individual nurses the recording week was not necessarily a 'typical' or 'average' week—indeed some were off sick or on leave for the whole week. However, when the whole sample of nurses of a particular type are considered as a group an accurate picture of an average week for that type of nurse is produced.

The nurses completed a page of the diary for each of the seven days (a blank diary page is shown on page 34). For each day a nurse first completed the top part of the page to show whether she was at work, off sick, off duty, etc., whether she was 'on call' and whether she was accompanied by anyone such as a student or supervisor. If she was 'on call', she recorded the total number of hours spent 'on call' that day.

The nurse recorded all her work activities in the main grid and if she was not at work that day the grid would normally be blank. Each time she moved from one location to another she completed a line of the diary and recorded information about the travelling time, the location, the amount of time spent there, the activities carried out and the time spent on each activity. Details about the client/patient were also recorded where applicable. The information was recorded using numerical codes.

The codes for the activities carried out fell into two broad categories—a) so called non-clinical activities which included telephone calls, meetings, clerical and administrative work and b) activities with clients/patients comprising technical, nursing and advisory activities. A list of the codes and of the activities which the codes represent is given in Chapter 9. Where a nurse had not specified what activity had been carried out although the time taken had been recorded, this has been classed as time on 'unspecified' activities. Examination of the diaries showed this to be most common where nurses were involved in clinics—they recorded, say, two hours spent doing an ante-natal clinic and felt that to be an adequate explanation of the activities performed. As the 'unspecified' activities seem more likely therefore to be activities with clients/patients than non-clinical ones they have been included in totals of time spent on activities with clients/patients.

Thus from the diary we have been able to calculate, for each nurse, the total working time during the week of diary completion and the total time spent on various activities and at various locations. Generally the total time spent on a particular activity or at a particular location has been summed for all nurses of a particular type and divided by the number or nurses of that type to produce an average (for all nurses of that type) of the total time spent on that activity or at that location.

6.4 Proportion of time spent on travel and other activities

The total number of hours worked by nurses during the week of diary recording can be divided into time spent travelling, time spent on non-clinical activities, time spent with clients/patients and time spend on activities which the nurse did not specify. Table 6.5 shows the proportion of the average total working time spent by each type of nurse working in the community on each of these four categories of activity. It is generally more useful to compare the proportions of time spent travelling rather than the actual amounts of time because there was so much variation between the different types of nurses in the number of hours worked. (See Chapter 7 for more details of the variation.) Figure 6.1 does, however, show the average number of hours spent on travel, non-clinical and patient-related activities; the small amounts of time spent on unspecified activities have been included in the time spent on activities with patients.

There was some variation in the amounts and proportions of time spent on travelling by the different types of nurses. Looking at Table 6.5 we can see that some nurses such as GP employed practice nurses, family planning nurses and clinic nurses spent very small proportions of their time travelling, as one would expect because their work tended to be clinic or practice based. Health visitors and school nurses, and their assistant nurses, spent smaller proportions of time on travelling—13% to 16%—compared with 22% to 24% for district nurses and midwives. Again this may be because their work is more clinic based than that of district nurses and midwives—most of the work of district nurses, in particular, is concerned with home visits and therefore involves a lot of travelling from house to house. There were no significant differences between the different types of district nurses or between district nurses and auxiliaries in the proportion of time spent on travel.

There was also variation in the proportion of time spent on the other categories of activity. The proportion of working time spent on non-clinical activities ranged from 16% for auxiliaries to 56% and 57% for liaison and GP employed practice nurses respectively. A high proportion of health visitors' average working time was spent on these activities—46%. Most types of nurses spent at least a quarter of their time on non-clinical activities—district nurse SENs and auxiliaries were the only exceptions. Non-clinical activities are discussed in detail in Chapter 10.

Table 6.5 Proportions of working time spent on travel, non-clinical and patient-related activities, by type of nurse

Travel and activities	All DNs	DN SRN+	DN SRN−	DN SEN+	DN SEN−	Auxil-iaries	GP empl.	Mid-wives	DN/ Midw.	HV	HV ass.	Schl. Nurse	Sch.N ass.	Fam. Plan.	Comm. Psych.	Geria-tric	Liai-son	Clinic
	%	%	%	%	%	%	%	%	%	%	%	%	%	%	%	%	%	%
Travel	24	24	24	26	25	21	3	22	23	16	13	13	13	5	21	20	17	8
Activities:																		
non-clinical	26	28	26	24	21	16	57	29	30	46	45	42	42	40	41	39	56	44
with patients	48	46	48	49	53	62	39	45	44	35	37	42	43	53	36	38	26	46
unspecified	2	2	2	1	1	1	1	4	3	3	5	3	2	2	2	3	1	2
Average hours worked per week (= 100%)	33.6	35.0	26.7	38.1	32.2	24.6	19.0	34.3	35.0	32.8	25.7	29.7	32.6	10.3	35.5	30.5	35.9	25.4
Number of nurses†	736	410	158	116	52	541	252	313	91	967	63	409	35	202	117	39	48	48

†Bases are smaller than on previous tables because this table, and all subsequent tables in this chapter, are based on information from the diaries. As explained in Chapter 1 some nurses were interviewed but did not complete the diary.

For each page RING DAY NUMBER ⟶

	Mon	Tues	Wed	Thur	Fri	Sat	Sun
	1	2	3	4	5	6	7

At the start
of each
new day
RECORD

(i)

	Whole day	Half day
At work	1	6
On annual leave	2	7
Off sick	3	8
On course/conference	4	9
Day off (for weekend & off-duty)	5	10

(iii)

Record whether accompanied by:

	Whole day	Part day/ session only
Student/pupil/trainee	1	5
Supervisor	2	6
Auxiliary	3	7
Other	4	8

(ii) On Call 1

12pm   6am   12noon   am

12noon   6pm   12pm   pm

TOTAL HOURS ON CALL [ ]

(iv) TIMING

TIME STARTED	TRAVEL TIME TO LOCATION	TIME AT LOCATION	LOCATION ⟶

LOCATION

(v) What ACTIVITIES did you carry out?

1		2		3		4		5	
CODE	TIME	CODE	TIME	CODE	TIME	CODE	TIME	CODE	TIME

ACTIVITIES

(vi) CLIENT/PATIENT DETAILS

AGE & SEX	HSEHLD TYPE	CLIENT TYPE	INITIATED BY

CLIENT/PATIENT

(vii) CLINIC/SESSIONS

CLINIC TYPE	NO. SEEN

CLINICS

34

Fig. 6.1 Average working time (hours) spent on travelling, non-clinical and patient-related activities by type of nurse

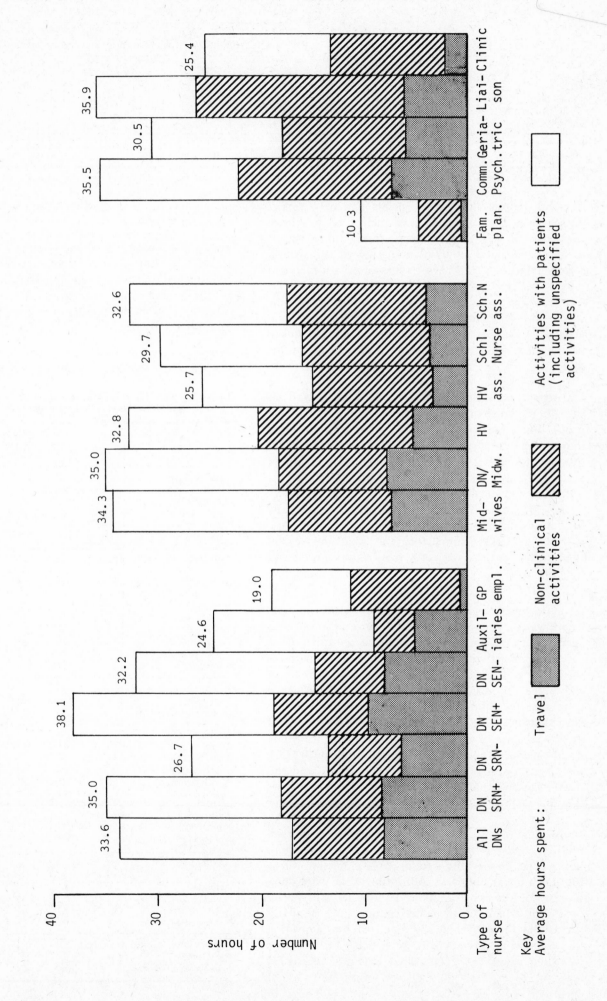

Key
Average hours spent:

Travel

Non-clinical activities

Activities with patients (including unspecified activities)

Table 6.6 Proportion of working time spent on travel, non-clinical and patient-related activities, by attachment

Travel and activities	District nurses		Midwives		Health visitors		Auxiliaries	
	Not attached	Attached	Not attached	Attached	Not attached	Attached	Not attached	Attached
	%	%	%	%	%	%	%	%
Travel	24	24	20	22	15	16	18	24
Activities								
non-clinical	29	27	31	29	48	46	21	13
with patients	46	48	46	45	34	35	60	62
unspecified	1	1	3	4	3	3	1	1
Average hours worked per week (= 100%)	27.4	35.6	34.7	35.4	31.5	33.3	24.6	25.1
Number of nurses†	*111*	*529*	*53*	*237*	*106*	*835*	*140*	*314*

†Full-time relief nurses, bath attendants and night sitters were not asked about attachment and so were not included in the table.

Turning to activities with clients/patients—district nurses spent just under half of their time on these. Auxiliaries spent the highest proportion of time—62%—with patients—and family planning nurses also spent a high proportion—53%. Most types of nurses recorded only a small percentage of working time for which the type of activity was unspecified. The proportions of time spent on non-clinical and unspecified activities and activities with patients are discussed in more detail in Chapter 9 in which travelling time is excluded from the tables.

The proportion of time spent on travel by nurses who felt they did too much or far too much was compared with the proportion for nurses who felt the amount of travelling they did was about right. Overall nurses who felt they did too much travelling spent a slightly higher proportion of time on travel—21% compared to 18%—but the difference was not significant. When the different types of nurses were looked at separately there were generally similar small non-significant differences between those with different views about their travelling. For several types of nurses there were only small numbers who said that their travelling was excessive, as seen in Table 6.2.

6.5 Attachment and proportion of time spent on travel

There was very little variation in the proportion of time spent on travel—or indeed on any of the other three categories of activity—for nurses with different patterns of working. Considering attachment first, Table 6.6 shows the proportions for attached and not attached district nurses, midwives, health visitors and auxiliaries. There was no variation except for auxiliaries—attached auxiliaries spent a greater proportion of time travelling and a smaller proportion of time on non-clinical work than those who were not attached. There were no differences between attached nurses with different types of attachment for any of these groups of nurses.

In Section 6.2 we saw that attached district nurses, midwives and health visitors were more likely than those not attached to view the amount of travelling they did as too much or far too much. According to the diary data, however, it was only the auxiliaries who actually spent a greater proportion of their time on travelling. Similarly we saw that those working additional patches or covering the whole of a GP area were more likely to view their travelling as excessive but there were no differences between them and nurses with other patterns of

attachment in the proportion of time which they actually spent on travelling.

Figure 6.2 shows the average number of hours spent on travel, non-clinical activities and activities with patients by attached and not attached district nurses, midwives, health visitors and auxiliaries. There is very little variation in even the number of hours spent on travelling and other activities.

Moving on to consider the number of practices nurses worked with, Table 6.7 shows that again there was very

Table 6.7 Proportion of working time spent on travel, non-clinical and patient-related activities, by number of practices worked with

Travel and activities	Number of practices			
	1	2	3–4	5+
District nurses	%	%	%	%
Travel	24	25	25	24
Activities:				
non-clinical	27	27	25	27
with patients	48	47	47	48
unspecified	1	1	3	1
Average hours worked per week (= 100%)	37.1	35.4	33.2	29.2
Number of district nurses	*288*	*126*	*90*	*108*
Midwives	%	%	%	%
Travel	23	21	22	20
Activities:				
non-clinical	29	31	27	30
with patients	44	45	46	46
unspecified	4	3	5	4
Average hours worked per week (= 100%)	36.2	35.7	34.9	36.6
Number of midwives	*53*	*74*	*72*	*81*
Health visitors	%	%	%	%
Travel	16	17	17	15
Activities:				
non-clinical	46	45	46	46
with patients	35	35	35	36
unspecified	3	3	2	3
Average hours worked per week (= 100%)	33.7	32.6	33.0	32.3
Number of health visitors	*559*	*179*	*80*	*103*
Auxiliaries	%	%	%	%
Travel	25	21	22	22
Activities:				
non-clinical	13	15	14	15
with patients	61	62	63	63
unspecified	1	2	1	*
Average hours worked per week (= 100%)	24.5	24.8	25.6	27.1
Number of auxiliaries	*160*	*85*	*75*	*48*

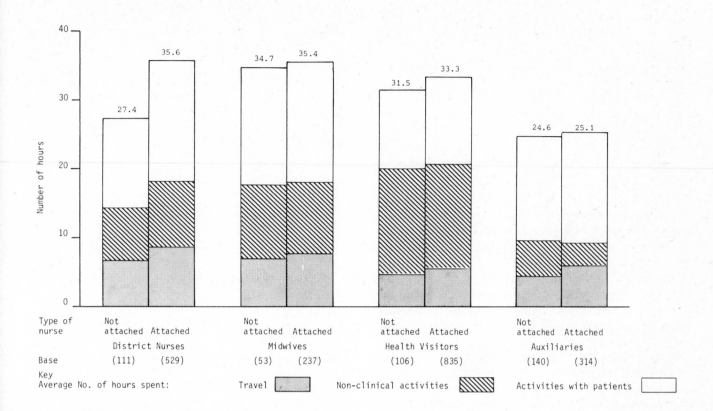

little variation in the proportion of time spent on travel, non-clinical and patient-related activities by nurses working with different numbers of practices, even among auxiliaries.

6.6 Proportion of activity time spent at different locations

Table 6.8 shows the proportion of activity time (that is, all time except travelling time) spent at different locations for the different types of nurses. District nurses, district nurse/midwives and auxiliaries spent the most time in patients' homes, with the SEN district nurses spending higher proportions of their time there than the SRNs. Within the district nursing service there was a trend for the less qualified staff to spend a larger proportion of the time in patients' homes than those with more qualifications. The percentages ranged from 58% for

district nurse SRNs with district training through 67% and 70% for district nurse SENs with and without a district nursing qualification respectively to 75% for auxiliaries.

District nurses, joint duty staff and midwives were the only nurses who spent much time working at home—14% of district nurses time and 21% of midwives time was spent at home. As seen in Chapter 3, high proportions of these types of nurses worked on a daily basis from home rather than from health centres, practice premises etc. Midwives spent 11% of their time in hospitals. This varied greatly depending on the different arrangements that health districts made for dividing midwifery between hospital and community.

Among the other nurses GP employed practices nurses, health visitors and assistants, family planning and clinic

Table 6.8 Proportion of activity time spent at different locations, by type of nurse

Location	All DNs	DN SRN+	DN SRN−	DN SEN+	DN SEN−	Auxil-iaries	GP empl.	Mid-wives	DN/ Midw.	HV	HV ass.	Schl. Nurse	Sch.N ass.	Fam. Plan.	Comm. Psych.	Geria-tric	Liai-son	Clinic
	%	%	%	%	%	%	%	%	%	%	%	%	%	%	%	%	%	%
Patient's home	60	58	59	67	70	75	2	46	55	28	18	5	2	2	35	46	17	8
Health premises†	20	22	17	16	16	13	89	20	19	53	57	37	44	64	11	42	18	66
Nurse's own home	14	15	14	14	11	6	2	21	22	5	2	4	2	2	4	5	6	1
Hospitals	3	2	5	1	1	1	*	11	1	4	5	1	*	16	41	4	52	10
Schools	*	*	*	–	*	2	–	–	–	2	10	47	48	2	1	–	1	4
Community premises††	*	*	*	1	*	1	1	*	*	3	3	1	1	*	2	*	*	1
Other locations	3	3	4	2	2	2	6	2	3	5	5	5	3	14	6	3	6	10
Average activity hours per week (= 100%)	25.5	26.8	20.2	28.4	24.0	19.4	22.4	26.9	27.2	27.5	22.4	25.9	28.4	9.8	28.1	24.5	29.8	23.2
Number of nurses	*736*	*410*	*158*	*116*	*52*	*541*	*252*	*313*	*91*	*967*	*63*	*409*	*35*	*202*	*117*	*39*	*48*	*48*

†Health premises include health centres, GP premises and AHA premises.
††Community premises include church/village halls, nurseries and day centres.

Table 6.9 Proportion of time spent at different locations by whether or not nurses were attached

Location	District nurses		Midwives		Health visitors		Auxiliaries	
	Not attached	Attached	Not attached	Attached	Not attached	Attached	Not attached	Attached
	%	%	%	%	%	%	%	%
Patient's home	59	60	41	46	24	29	65	81
Health premises†	15	21	13	22	48	54	21	9
Nurse's own home	13	15	19	22	5	5	5	8
Hospital	8	2	25	8	10	3	1	*
School	–	*	*	*	4	1	3	*
Community premises††	*	*	*	*	2	3	1	1
Off-duty and other	5	2	2	2	7	5	4	1
Average activity hours per week (= 100%)	20.7	27.1	27.7	27.8	26.9	27.9	20.1	19.1
Number of nurses	*111*	*529*	*53*	*237*	*106*	*835*	*140*	*314*

†Health premises include health centres, GP premises and AHA premises.
††Community premises include church/village halls, nurseries and day centres.

nurses all spent more than half of their time at health premises. School nurses and assistants spent almost half of their time, not surprisingly, in schools and around two fifths of their time at health premises. At hospitals, liaison nurses spent 52% of their time there and community psychiatric nurses 41% although the latter also spent 35% of their time in patients' homes. Geriatric nurses' time was mainly split between patients' homes and health premises.

There was some variation in the proportion of time spent at different locations by attachment and number of practices. Table 6.9 shows the differences between the attached and those who were not attached for the four main types of nurses. Attached district nurses spent a higher proportion of time at health premises and a lower proportion at hospitals than district nurses who were not attached although the differences were small. These findings also applied to midwives although the differences were much larger—not attached midwives spent 25% of their time in hospitals compared with 8% for attached midwives; the corresponding proportions for health premises were 13% and 22%. This probably reflects the different locations of ante-natal clinics. Attached health visitors tended to spend a greater proportion of their time at health premises and clients' homes and less in hospitals that those who were not attached but again the differences were small. The pattern was clearer for auxiliaries with attached staff spending 81% of their time in patients' homes compared to 64% for those not attached. The latter spent much more of their time (23%) at health premises than the attached auxiliaries (9%)—the reverse of the trend for the other three types of nurses.

The proportion of time spent at different locations by nurses working with different numbers of practices was also examined. There was no clear pattern of variation. District nurses who worked with larger numbers of practices tended to spend less time at health premises and midwives and health visitors who worked with five or more practices spent a greater proportion of their time at hospitals. There was no significant variation for auxiliaries. The number of practices worked with was not related to the proportion of time spent in patients' homes for any of the four types of nurse.

Table 6.10 shows the proportion of time spent at the various locations by nurses with different daily work

Table 6.10 Proportion of time spent at different locations by nurse's daily work base

Location	Work base			
	Home	Health premises†	Hospital	Other††
District nurses	%	%	%	%
Patient's home	61	61	50	53
Health premises	18	24	5	31
Nurses' home	17	11	5	8
Hospital	1	1	33	3
School	*	*	–	*
Community premises	*	*	1	*
Other	3	3	6	5
Average activity hours per week (= 100%)	26.1	26.3	19.9	20.8
Number of nurses	*465*	*189*	*35*	*42*
Midwives	%		%	
Patient's home	47	(11.4)	31	–
Health premises	22	(7.8)	5	–
Nurses' home	20	(4.3)	10	–
Hospital	9	(0.3)	51	–
School	*	–	–	–
Community premises	*	(0.1)	–	–
Other	2	(1.2)	3	–
Average activity hours per week (= 100%)	26.8	25.1	29.3	0.0
Number of nurses	*277*	*16*	*20*	*0*
Health visitors	%	%	%	%
Patient's home	33	28	20	31
Health premises	27	56	14	51
Nurses' home	25	4	5	4
Hospital	4	3	50	2
School	2	1	2	2
Community premises	4	3	1	5
Other	5	5	8	5
Average activity hours per week (= 100%)	26.1	27.7	29.7	23.0
Number of nurses	*58*	*847*	*21*	*41*
Auxiliaries	%	%		%
Patient's home	84	54	(8.0)	56
Health premises	6	33	(0.3)	18
Nurses' home	8	5	(2.9)	*
Hospital	*	*	(1.8)	1
School	*	3	–	18
Community premises	*	2	(0.3)	–
Other	2	3	–	7
Average activity hours per week (= 100%)	19.8	19.4	13.3	18.5
Number of nurses	*366*	*138*	*14 ø*	*21*

† Health premises includes clinics, health centres and practice premises.
†† Other includes community health offices, schools and other bases.
ø Base was too small for percentages to be calculated.

bases. The most striking but obvious differences occurred between those based in hospital and those based elsewhere. For example hospital based community midwives spent one half of their time in hospital compared with less than one tenth by home based midwives. However very few of any of the nurses working in the community were based in hospitals. There were the expected differences between staff based at home and in health premises. These were particularly pronounced among health visitors and auxiliaries.

7 Hours worked and 'on call' time

7.1 Number of hours worked

Table 7.1 shows, for each type of nurse, the average number of working hours recorded for the entire week and the distribution of nurses working different numbers of hours.

There were large differences between the different types of nurses in the average hours worked. District nurse SENs with a district nursing qualification had the highest average hours, 38.1. Family planning nurses worked the least hours on average—10.3 hours—followed by GP employed practice nurses with 19 hours. Auxiliaries, clinic nurses, health visitor assistants and district nurse SRNs without a district nursing qualification all had relatively low average hours ranging from 24.6 to 26.7 hours. All these six types of nurses had large numbers working part-time (see Chapter 3). This accounts for the low average hours worked—62% of family planning nurses, for example, worked for less than 11 hours.

Table 7.2 compares the hours worked during the week of diary recording with the average weekly hours as reported in the interview†. All nurses gave an answer to this question but of course during the recording week a small proportion of nurses worked no hours because of sickness or annual leave. These have been omitted from part a) of the table. As can be seen the distributions at a) and b) are different for each nurse type. Part b) of the table shows the individual nurse's average working hours which probably reflect their contracted hours. These figures are also useful for distinguishing those who worked full or part-time and those who commonly reported working more than 40 hours a week. Part b) is an extension of Table 3.1 and full and part-time working is discussed in Chapter 3. Compared with part b) of Table 7.2 the hours worked in part a) are more widely spread. This is because they reflect the actual hours worked in one week. Some nurses would have worked fewer than their average hours because of odd days sickness or leave—others would have worked more than their average hours covering for absent colleagues. In addition the diary record also included

---

†Question 13 (Excluding 'on call' time) How many hours on average do you work in a week?

Table 7.1 Hours worked during the week's diary recording, by type of nurse

Hours worked	All DNs	DN SRN+	DN SRN-	DN SEN+	DN SEN-	Auxil-iaries	GP empl.	Mid-wives	DN/ Midw.	HV	HV ass.	Schl. Nurse	Sch.N ass.	Fam. Plan.	Comm. Psych.	Geria-tric	Liai-son	Clinic
	%	%	%	%	%	%	%	%	%	%	%	%	%	%	%	%	%	%
None	5	4	7	5	1	4	4	3	-	2	2	2	6	7	4	5	-	2
Up to 10	6	5	12	2	4	9	22	7	9	4	5	5	6	55	1	3	2	12
11 – 20	11	9	20	6	17	23	34	9	9	10	27	18	-	25	6	23	15	31
21 – 30	17	15	21	14	18	35	20	21	14	21	36	23	11	9	20	18	12	14
31 – 40	28	31	19	30	27	18	17	25	26	35	20	37	54	2	26	15	40	23
41 – 49	21	23	19	30	21	9	2	18	31	24	8	12	23	2	35	33	23	16
50+	12	13	9	13	12	2	1	17	11	4	2	3	-	*	8	3	8	2
Average total hours worked	33.6	35.0	26.7	38.1	32.2	24.6	19.0	34.3	35.0	32.8	25.7	29.7	32.6	10.3	35.5	30.5	35.9	25.4
Number of nurses (= 100%)	736	410	158	116	52	541	252	313	91	967	63	409	35	202	117	39	48	48

Table 7.2 A comparison of weekly hours worked, as recorded in the diary and questionnaire, by type of nurse

Assessment	All DNs	DN SRN+	DN SRN-	DN SEN+	DN SEN-	Auxil-iaries	GP empl.	Mid-wives	DN/ Midw.	HV	HV ass.	Schl. Nurse	Sch.N ass.	Fam. Plan.	Comm. Psych.	Geria-tric	Liai-son	Clinic
(a) Diary	%	%	%	%	%	%	%	%	%	%	%	%	%	%	%	%	%	%
Up to 10	6	5	13	2	4	9	23	7	9	4	5	5	6	59	1	3	2	12
11 – 20	12	9	21	6	17	24	35	9	9	10	28	18	-	27	6	24	15	32
21 – 30	18	16	23	15	18	37	21	22	14	21	37	24	12	10	21	19	12	14
31 – 40	29	32	20	32	28	19	18	26	26	36	20	38	57	2	27	16	40	24
41 – 49	22	24	13	32	21	9	2	19	31	25	8	12	25	2	37	35	23	16
50+	13	14	10	13	12	2	1	17	11	4	2	3	-	*	8	3	8	2
Average total hours worked	35.4	36.5	28.7	40.1	32.5	25.6	19.8	35.4	35.0	33.5	26.2	30.3	34.7	11.1	37.0	32.1	35.9	25.9
Number of nurses (= 100%)	699	394	147	110	51	519	242	304	91	948	62	401	33	188	112	37	48	47
(b) Questionnaire																		
Up to 10	4	2	14	-	3	4	12	2	-	1	2	-	-	57	-	-	-	4
11 – 20	9	4	23	2	19	41	39	5	1	7	33	17	7	30	1	13	10	31
21 – 30	5	4	9	4	3	22	23	3	4	9	22	32	9	8	1	14	4	17
31 – 40	69	74	48	81	69	33	24	73	70	70	43	49	79	3	64	57	70	48
41 – 49	11	13	6	13	5	*	1	13	18	12	-	2	5	1	28	16	16	-
50+	2	3	*	-	1	-	1	4	7	1	-	-	-	1	6	-	-	-
Number of nurses (= 100%)	824	457	171	132	64	609	291	371	102	1057	67	442	42	221	136	44	50	52

those hours actually worked when 'on call' whereas the question posed in the interview specifically excluded 'on call' time. However there was a tendency for nurses to record more hours in their diaries than their average reported hours suggested. One explanation may be the amount of non-clinical work that many nurses carry out in their own homes.† They may not have considered this when answering the average working hours in the interview.

7.2 Number of days worked

Table 7.3 shows the number of days worked during the week of diary recording by the different types of nurses working in the community. Around two fifths of many of the types of nurses—district nurses, midwives, joint duty district nurse/midwives, health visitors, school, geriatric and liaison nurses—had worked on five or more days of the week recorded. Some nurses worked on fewer than five days because of leave, sickness and training courses. The types of nurses where high proportions worked on less than five days were those who more often worked part-time, such as auxiliaries, GP employed practice nurses and family planning nurses. District nurse SRNs without a district nursing qualification worked on fewer

† See Chapter 10

days than other district nurses—they were also identified earlier as a group with a high proportion of part-timers and relief staff. Only district nurses, midwives and joint duty district nurse/midwives had sizeable proportions who had worked on six or seven days—26% of midwives and district nurse SENs with district training had done so.

Table 7.4 shows the proportions of the average time worked on weekdays and at weekends. From this it is clear that only district nurses, midwives and joint duty staff carried out more than a small proportion of their work at weekends. Twenty per cent of the average hours of midwives and district nurse/midwives were worked at the weekend and 14% of all district nurses.

Table 7.5 shows the proportions of nurses who had time away from work, because of either sickness or leave. Overall four per cent of nurses working in the community were off sick for one day or more during the period of diary recording. A much higher proportion of nurses, 20% overall, had at least one day's leave during the period.

7.3 Hours worked by attachment and number of practices worked with

Table 7.6 shows, using the information from the questionnaire, that a higher proportion of not attached district nurses than attached nurses were part-timers—

Table 7.3 Number of days worked, by type of nurse

Number of days	All DNs	DN SRN+	DN SRN–	DN SEN+	DN SEN–	Auxil-iaries	GP empl.	Mid-wives	DN/Midw.	HV	HV ass.	Schl. Nurse	Sch.N ass.	Fam. Plan.	Comm. Psych.	Geria-tric	Liai-son	Clinic
	%	%	%	%	%	%	%	%	%	%	%	%	%	%	%	%	%	%
None	7	6	12	5	4	8	10	5	5	3	5	3	9	30	5	8	–	7
One	8	6	16	4	8	13	17	7	7	6	4	7	3	46	2	3	5	15
Two	11	10	17	4	15	42	36	11	11	13	27	15	3	16	15	11	16	22
Three	12	11	14	13	13	13	15	14	14	15	32	16	6	4	14	27	14	15
Four	25	28	19	22	23	7	13	23	23	20	10	21	–	2	24	8	20	11
Five	20	22	12	26	23	16	9	14	26	43	22	38	76	2	39	38	45	30
Six	16	16	10	25	14	1	–	20	14	*	–	*	3	–	1	5	–	–
Seven	1	1	–	1	–	*	–	6	–	–	–	–	–	–	–	–	–	–
Number of nurses (= 100%)†	699	390	152	108	49	487	229	300	81	893	59	381	33	179	110	37	44	46
Average number of days worked	3.7	3.8	2.9	4.3	3.7	2.5	2.3	4.0	3.8	3.7	3.0	3.6	4.2	1.1	3.7	3.6	3.8	3.0

†Bases are smaller than usual because some nurses had not always recorded whether or not they were at work and they were excluded from the analysis

Table 7.4 Proportion of hours worked on weekdays and weekends, by type of nurse

Time of the week	All DNs	DN SRN+	DN SRN–	DN SEN+	DN SEN–	Auxil-iaries	GP empl.	Mid-wives	DN/Midw.	HV	HV ass.	Schl. Nurse	Sch.N ass.	Fam. Plan.	Comm. Psych.	Geria-tric	Liai-son	Clinic
	%	%	%	%	%	%	%	%	%	%	%	%	%	%	%	%	%	%
Weekdays	86	86	84	84	89	96	96	80	80	99	100	99	100	97	98	96	99	99
Weekend	14	14	16	16	11	4	4	20	20	1	*	1	*	3	2	4	1	1
Average hours worked per week (=100%)	33.6	35.0	26.7	38.1	32.2	24.6	19.0	34.3	35.0	32.8	25.7	29.7	32.6	10.3	35.5	30.5	35.9	25.4
Number of nurses	736	410	158	116	52	541	252	313	91	967	63	409	35	202	117	39	48	48

Table 7.5 Days away from work, by type of nurse

Reasons for absence	All DNs	DN SRN+	DN SRN–	DN SEN+	DN SEN–	Auxil-iaries	GP empl.	Mid-wives	DN/midw.	HV	HV ass.	Schl. Nurse	Sch.N ass.	Fam. Plan.	Comm. Psych.	Geria-tric	Liai-son	Clinic
Nurses who had one day or more:																		
off sick	3%	3%	3%	6%	2%	5%	4%	4%	4%	4%	5%	6%	6%	3%	6%	8%	9%	2%
on leave	20%	22%	15%	20%	12%	15%	14%	22%	23%	25%	17%	15%	6%	8%	34%	27%	30%	15%
Number of nurses (=100%)†	699	390	152	108	49	487	229	300	81	893	59	381	33	179	110	37	44	46

† Bases are smaller than usual because some nurses had not always recorded whether or not they were at work and they were excluded from the analysis

42% compared with 9%. However for the other three types of nurses differences were either very small or non-existent. There were no differences for any of the nurses between those working different types of attachment.

Table 7.7 shows the average hours worked recorded in the diaries by district nurses, midwives, health visitors and auxiliaries according to whether or not they were attached to general practice. There was very little difference between the attached and not attached nurses except for district nurses—attached district nurses worked an average of 35.6 hours compared with 27.4 hours for those who were not attached. As we have just seen district nurses who were not attached were more likely to work part-time than those who were attached.

There were no differences in the average hours worked by nurses with different patterns of attachment for any of the four types of nurses.

Table 7.8 shows the average hours worked by the same types of nurses according to the number of practices they worked with. Again district nurses showed the clearest trend; the average number of hours worked was lower the

greater the number of practices worked with. There was no clear pattern for midwives and health visitors. For auxiliaries the average hours worked were generally higher for nurses who worked with more practices, but the differences were not large.

Table 7.8 Average hours worked by nurses working with different numbers of practices

	Number of practices worked with			
	1	2	3-4	5+
District nurses				
Average hours worked	37.1	35.4	33.2	29.2
Number of district nurses	288	126	90	108
Midwives				
Average hours worked	36.2	35.7	34.9	36.6
Number of midwives	53	74	72	81
Health visitors				
Average hours worked	33.7	32.6	33.0	32.3
Number of health visitors	559	179	80	103
Auxiliaries				
Average hours worked	24.5	24.8	25.6	27.1
Number of auxiliaries	160	85	75	48

Table 7.6 Full and part-time working, by type of attachment

	Not attached	Attached			Attached		
		All parts	Specific parts	All + patch	Specific + patch	All attached
District nurses	%	%	%	%	%	%
Part-time	42	9	5	12	9	9
Full-time	58	91	95	88	91	91
Number of district nurses (= 100%)	126	336	87	105	66	594
Midwives	%	%		%	%	%
Part-time	12	7	(–)	8	4	6
Full-time	88	93	(18)	92	96	94
Number of midwives (= 100%)	66	114	18†	97	54	283
Health visitors	%	%	%	%	%	%
Part-time	11	15	15	12	21	16
Full-time	89	85	85	88	79	84
Number of health visitors (= 100%)	120	380	282	120	132	914
Auxiliaries	%	%	%	%	%	%
Part-time	65	67	64	55	46	64
Full-time	35	33	36	45	54	36
Number of auxiliaries (= 100%)	162	227	62	38	26	353

† Percentages have not been calculated because the base is too small. Actual numbers are given in brackets

Table 7.7 Average hours worked, by attached and not attached nurses

	District nurses		Midwives		Health visitors		Auxiliaries	
	Not attached	Attached	Not attached	Attached	Not attached	Attached	Not attached	Attached
Average hours worked per week	27.4	35.7	34.7	35.4	31.5	33.3	24.6	25.1
Number of nurses	111	529	53	237	106	835	140	314

7.4 'On call' duty

In the interview nurses were asked 'Do you do any 'on call' duty?' Only very small proportions of some kinds of nurses working in the community did any 'on call' duty. Table 7.9 shows that just over a tenth of community psychiatric, geriatric and liaison nurses did 'on call' duty. One half of the district nurses did some and nearly all the midwives and joint duty district nurse/midwives did 'on call' duty. District nurses with district training were more likely to do 'on call' duty than those without. Looking just at district nurses, midwives and joint duty staff, few worked part-time, but those who did were much less likely than full-time staff to do any 'on call' duty—26% compared with 70%.

Table 7.10 uses diary information to show the proportions of nurses who record time spent 'on call' in addition to the hours worked. Health visitor assistants and school nurse assistants did no 'on call' duty and only very small proportions of some other types of nurses did any. On the other hand, about three quarters of midwives and district nurse/midwives did some 'on call' duty, as did 40% of district nurses. Among district nurses those with a district nursing qualification were more likely to have done some 'on call' duty than those without.

There was a large variation in the average number of hours spent 'on call' for those nurses who had done some 'on call' duty. District nurses, midwives and joint duty staff had high levels of 'on call' duty and amongst the district nurses it was the district nurse SRNs, both with and without district training, who spent most hours 'on call'. Some nurses, such as health visitors and liaison nurses, had very high average hours 'on call' due to small proportions of nurses spending a lot of time 'on call'.

Those types of nurses with high proportions recording 'on call' duty in their diaries generally reported a high incidence of 'on call' duty at the interview (see Table 7.9). However, the proportions who reported doing 'on call' duty at the interview were higher than those shown in Table 7.10. The interview question asked whether nurses did *any* 'on call' duty whereas the diary information recorded 'on call' duty during the week of diary completion only. During the diary week some nurses would not have had to do any 'on call' work, others would have been off sick or on leave.

Table 7.11 shows the proportions of nurses who recorded time spent 'on call' on weekdays and the weekend. Only among district nurses, midwives and joint duty staff were substantial proportions 'on call' at the weekend. These were also the only types of nurses who carried out more than a small part of their work at weekends.

The average number of hours 'on call' on weekdays is usually greater than the average number of hours 'on call' at weekends but as the average for weekdays could have been spread over a maximum of five days whereas the weekend average covered at most two days, the average number of hours 'on call' per day is probably higher at the weekend than for weekdays.

The numbers of nurses doing 'on call' duty was insufficient to examine the relationships between 'on call' work and different situations, such as attachment and number of practices worked with.

Table 7.9 Incidence of 'on call' duty, by type of nurse

Whether nurse does 'on call' duty	ALL DNs	DN SRN+	DN SRN-	DN SEN+	DN SEN-	Auxil- iaries	GP empl.	Mid- wives	DN/ Midw.	HV	HV ass.	Schl. Nurse	Sch.N ass.	Fam. Plan.	Comm. Psych.	Geri- atric	Liai- son	Clinic
	%	%	%	%	%	%	%	%	%	%	%	%	%	%	%	%	%	%
Yes	52	59	39	49	36	2	6	83	89	3	–	1	–	1	11	16	14	2
No	48	41	61	51	64	98	94	17	11	97	100	99	100	99	89	84	86	98
Number of nurses (= 100%)	824	457	171	132	64	609	291	371	102	1057	67	442	42	221	136	44	50	52

Table 7.10 'On call' duty recorded, by type of nurse

Whether nurse recorded any 'on call' duty	All DNs	DN SRN+	DN SRN-	DN SEN+	DN SEN-	Auxil- iaries	GP empl.	Mid- wives	DN/ Midw.	HV	HV ass.	Schl. Nurse	Sch.N ass.	Fam. Plan.	Comm. Psych.	Geria- tric	Liai- son	Clinic
	%	%	%	%	%	%	%	%	%	%	%	%	%	%	%	%	%	%
Yes	40	45	30	39	31	4	8	73	77	2	–	1	–	2	1	13	6	2
No	60	55	70	61	69	96	92	27	23	98	100	99	100	98	99	87	94	98
Number of nurses (=100%)	736	410	158	116	52	541	252	313	91	967	63	409	35	202	117	39	48	48
Average hours 'on call' for those nurses who did any	21.4	23.6	21.4	13.9	14.6	22.8	34.0	34.7	36.0	87.9	0	24.5	0	5.1	0.1	7.0	51.2	14.7
Number of nurses 'on call'	295	186	47	46	16	20	20	228	70	22	0	5	0	4	1	5	3	1

Table 7.11 Weekday and weekend 'on call' duty, by type of nurse

Weekday/weekend	All DNs	DN SRN+	DN SRN-	DN SEN+	DN SEN-	Auxil- iaries	GP Empl.	Mid- wives	DN/ Midw.	HV	HV ass.	Schl. Nurse	Sch.N ass.	Fam. Plan.	Comm. Psych.	Geria- tric	Liai- son	Clinic
Percentage of nurses 'on call' on weekdays	35%	41%	25%	32%	21%	3%	7%	71%	73%	2%	–	1%	–	2%	1%	10%	4%	2%
Average hours 'on call' on weekdays	17.4	18.7	18.1	11.6	13.4	21.2	27.6	26.0	27.7	63.0	–	17.2	–	3.7	4.0	7.5	47.0	15.0
Percentage of nurses 'on call' at weekend	18%	20%	14%	17%	13%	1%	3%	36%	37%	1%	–	*	–	–	–	3%	4%	–
Average hours 'on call' at the weekend	13.8	14.8	13.9	10.0	12.9	20.2	22.0	18.9	20.3	42.2	–	20.0	–	–	–	5.0	30.0	–
Number of nurses (=100%)	736	410	158	116	58	541	252	313	91	697	63	409	35	202	117	39	48	48

8 Patients/clients cared for by nurses working in the community

8.1 Description of the information about patients recorded in the diaries

When a nurse carried out or assisted at a clinic or GP surgery session she recorded the type of clinic and the total number of patients seen but did not record details about each individual patient. When making home visits, however, or seeing individual patients at any other location the nurse recorded information about each patient: this included the patient's age and sex, the patient's household type, who initiated the visit or contact and the type of patient—diabetic, hospital discharge, etc. The information about both clinics and individual patients was recorded using numerical codes and a list of the codes and the details they represented is shown below.

CLIENT/PATIENT DETAILS

AGE AND SEX

01	Up to 1	
02	1-4	child
03	5-15	

11	16-19	
12	20-29	
13	30-44	
14	45-54	
15	55-64	woman
16	65-74	
17	75-84	
18	85+	

21	16-19	
22	20-29	
23	30-44	
24	45-54	
25	55-64	man
26	65-74	
27	75-84	
28	85+	

31	Children	
32	Young & middle aged adults	
33	The elderly	Groups
34	Whole family	
35	Other mixtures (specify)	

HOUSEHOLD TYPE

01 Does not apply—not home visit
02 Lone adult—with or without children
03 Adults only—all aged 65+
04 All other household types
05 Don't know

WHO INITIATED THIS CONTACT

01 Primary visit to new born baby
02 Yourself—first visit
03 Yourself—routine, follow-up
04 Client/patient or their family
05 GP
06 Other member of practice team
07 Other community nursing staff
08 Hospital
09 School health service/teacher
10 Social services staff
11 Voluntary agency/worker
12 No-one ie chance meeting
13 Other (specify)

TYPE OF CLIENT/PATIENT

01 Expectant mother
02 Maternity—within 28 days of delivery
03 Baby, toddler or child and person caring for it
04 Schoolchild and/or person caring for it
05 Post-operative, hospital discharge (last 28 days)
06 Terminal/deteriorating
07 Physical handicap also inc. arthritis, rheumatism, paralysis other limitations on mobility etc.
08 Mental handicap, subnormality
09 Mental illness inc. depression, senile dementia, confusion personality disorder etc.
10 Chest disease inc. TB, bronchitis, pneumonia and infections etc.
11 Cardio-vascular disease inc. heart, stroke and hypertension patients
12 Skin inc. ulcers, pressure sores, etc.
13 Diabetic
14 Elderly—general frailty or no specific condition or condition not known
15 Other medical/surgical (specify)
16 Group visit eg. old people's home, community groups inc. wardens
17 Problem family
18 Other (specify)

TYPE OF CLINIC SESSION

01 Ante-natal and post-natal inc. relaxation, psychoprophylaxis and booking clinic
02 Well baby, infant welfare, child health
03 Developmental assessment
04 Immunisation and vaccination
05 Rubella vaccination
06 Mothercraft/parentcraft
07 Family planning
08 Well woman, cytology
09 Hearing and vision
10 School medicals/hygiene inspection
11 Health education sessions
12 GP surgery sessions
13 Other (specify)

Throughout this chapter, time spent with patients or in clinics is time spent on technical, nursing and advisory activities. When nurses carried out non-clinical activities they were not asked to record patient details although certain non-clinical activities (particularly telephone calls) may have, in some cases, involved patients. A number of nurses who completed the diary felt that telephone calls with patients should have been recorded separately, giving details about the patient, but at the pilot trial nurses had found it very difficult to separate calls with or about patients from other telephone calls. The recording of several items of information about each patient spoken to on the telephone was an additional problem. Therefore our estimates of time spent with patients do not include time spent talking to patients on the telephone. The time nurses spent making telephone calls will be considered in more detail in Chapter 10 which concentrates on non-clinical activity.

8.2 Proportion of time spent in clinics and home visits

Table 8.1 shows the proportions of their time with patients that the different types of nurses spent on clinics, home visits and other patient contacts. Clinics and home visits accounted for the majority of time spent with patients for most types of nurses. Figure 8.1 shows the average number of hours that the nurses spent on these three areas.

District nurses spent most of their time with patients making home visits—89% overall—with SEN district nurses spending a higher proportion of their time on this than the SRNs. Auxiliaries and district nurse/midwives also spent high proportions—92% and 85% respectively—of their time on home visits. All these types of nurses spent a small proportion of their time with patients doing clinics, with district nurse/midwives spending the largest proportion, 10%.

Midwives and health visitors spent a greater proportion of their time on clinics than the types of nurses mentioned in the previous paragraph—19% and 26% respectively—but both still spent more than half of their time making home visits. Health visitor assistants however, spent only 34% of their time on home visits and more, 43%, on clinics.

GP employed nurses, school, family planning and clinic nurses all spend a large proportion of their time—60% or more—doing clinics. Community psychiatric and geriatric nurses spent a large proportion of their time with patients on home visits.

'Other' patient contacts mainly involved time spent with individual patients in other locations, such as health premises, hospitals and schools. Only school nurse assistants spent more than half (59%) of their time with patients on other patient contacts—mainly with children in schools. Liaison nurses spent 39% of their time on other patient contacts, usually with individual patients in hospitals.

There was some variation in the proportions of time spent on clinics, home visits and other patient contacts by nurses with different working patterns. Looking first at attachment, Table 8.2 shows the proportions for attached and not attached district nurses, midwives, health visitors and auxiliaries. Attached auxiliaries spent a greater proportion of their time on home visits than auxiliaries who were not attached. There were indications of a similar pattern for midwives and health visitors, with the attached nurses spending a corresponding lower proportion of time on 'other' patient contacts, but the differences were not significant. There were no differences between nurses working with different numbers of practices.

Looking again at Table 8.1 and Figure 8.1 it is clear that some types of nurses spent only a small *proportion* of their time and a small *amount* of time on clinics. District

Table 8.1 Proportion of time with patients spent on clinics and home visits, by type of nurse

Type of contact with patients	All DNs	DN SRN+	DN SRN−	DN SEN+	DN SEN−	Auxil-iaries	GP empl.	Mid-wives	DN/ Midw.	HV	HV ass.	Schl. Nurse	Sch.N ass.	Fam. Plan.	Comm. Psych.	Geria-tric	Liai-son	Clinic
	%	%	%	%	%	%	%	%	%	%	%	%	%	%	%	%	%	%
Clinics	5	7	6	3	2	4	60	19	10	26	43	66	38	70	8	3	17	61
Home visits	89	88	86	94	93	92	4	66	85	56	34	7	3	3	70	86	44	15
Other eg hospitals, schools	6	5	8	3	5	4	36	15	5	18	23	27	59	27	22	11	39	24
Average hours spent with patients (=100%)	16.6	16.9	13.2	19.3	17.4	15.4	7.7	16.9	16.6	12.5	10.6	13.5	15.0	5.6	13.4	12.6	9.8	12.2
Number of nurses	736	410	158	116	52	541	252	313	91	967	63	409	35	202	117	39	48	48

Table 8.2 Proportion of time spent with patients on clinics and home visits, by attached and not attached nurses

Type of patient contact	District nurses		Midwives		Health visitors		Auxiliaries	
	Not attached	Attached	Not attached	Attached	Not attached	Attached	Not attached	Attached
	%	%	%	%	%	%	%	%
Clinics	3	6	16	20	25	26	8	1
Home visits	90	89	62	66	50	58	86	96
Other, eg hospitals, schools	7	5	22	14	25	16	6	3
Average hours spent with patients (=100%)	12.9	17.6	17.0	17.5	11.7	12.7	15.0	15.8
Number of nurses	111	529	53	237	106	835	140	314

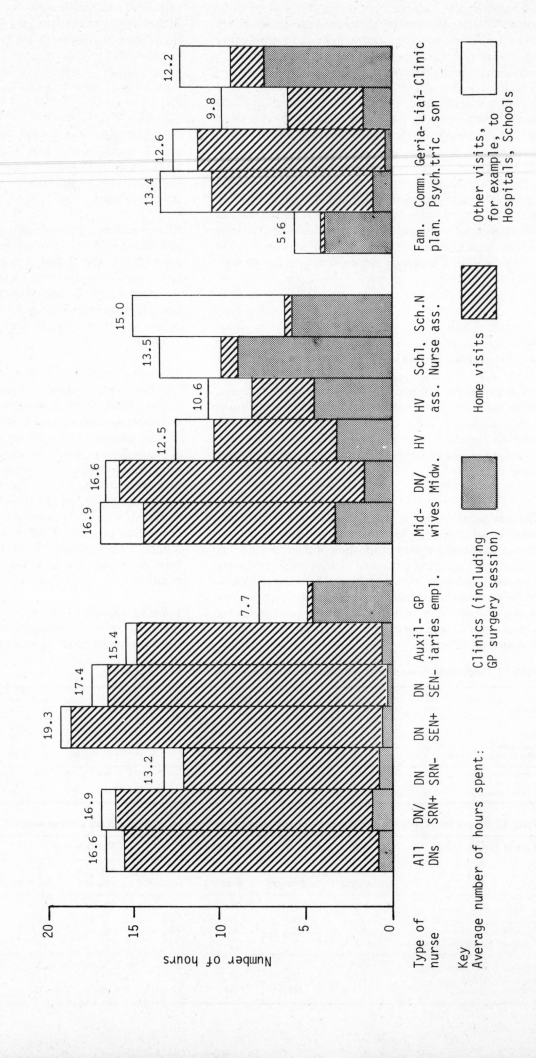

Fig. 8.1 Average time (hours) spent with patients in clinics, on home visits and other visits by type of nurse

Type of nurse: All DNs, DN/SRN+, DN SRN−, DN SEN+, DN SEN−, Auxil-iaries, GP empl., Mid-wives, DN/Midw., HV, HV Sch.N ass., Schl. Nurse ass., Fam. plan., Comm. Psych.tric, Geria-tric son, Liai-Clinic

Number of hours

Key
Average number of hours spent:

Clinics (including GP surgery session)

Home visits

Other visits, for example, to Hospitals, Schools

Values: 16.6, 16.9, 13.2, 19.3, 17.4, 15.4, 7.7, 16.9, 16.6, 12.5, 10.6, 13.5, 15.0, 5.6, 13.4, 12.6, 9.8, 12.2

nurses, auxiliaries, community psychiatric and geriatric nurses all spent less than 10% of their time and no more than 1.2 hours on average per week carrying out or assisting at clinics so they have been excluded from any further analysis of clinics. Similarly the types of nurses who spent much of their time on clinics and less than 10% on home visits have been excluded from further analysis on individual patient details. They are GP employed nurses, school nurses and assistants and family planning nurses.

8.3 Proportion of time spent on different types of clinics

Table 8.3 shows the time spent on different types of clinics as a proportion of the time spent on all clinics for the relevant types of nurses. Midwives and district nurse/midwives were mainly concerned with ante-natal and post-natal clinic sessions although joint duty district nurse/midwives also spent 29% of their clinic time on GP surgery sessions. District nurses are not shown on the table but most of the small amount of their clinic time was spent on GP surgery sessions. The joint duty district nurse/midwives were therefore probably doing GP surgery sessions as part of their district nurse duties.

Health visitors and assistants were particularly concerned with well baby, infant welfare and child health clinics, spending 54% and 25% respectively of their clinic time on this. School nurses and assistants spent most of their clinic time on school medicals, hygiene inspections and hearing and vision clinics and health visitor assistants also spent 23% of their clinic time on these kinds of clinics.

GP employed nurses spent only three quarters of their clinic time on GP surgery sessions, the other quarter being divided among many other types of clinics. Clinic nurses spent almost half of their time on GP surgery sessions. Liaison nurses mainly did 'other' clinics which probably specifically concerned liaison work and were not catered for by the specified codes.

Table 8.3 also shows the average number of patients seen in clinics during the week of diary recording for the different types of nurses. School nurses and assistants saw

the most patients and clinic nurses also had a high average. District nurse/midwives and liaison nurses spent less time than the other nurses on clinics and saw the fewest patients.

The average number of minutes spent with a clinic patient was calculated (by dividing the average time spent on all clinics by the number of patients seen) and is shown on the table. Liaison nurses had the highest average with 11 minutes whilst school nurses and assistants had the lowest averages—four and three minutes respectively with each clinic patient.

Section 8.3 looked at the time spent with patients in clinics. The next three sections look at the rest of the time spent with patients, that is time spent with individual patients either on home visits or in other locations.

8.4 Proportion of time spent with patients in different age and sex groups

Table 8.4 shows the proportion of time spent with patients in different age and sex groups for the relevant types of nurses. All types of nurses spent a greater proportion of their time with female patients than with male patients, often more than twice as much. Only clinic nurses spent almost equal proportions of their time with male and female patients—42% and 44% respectively.

Looking first at district nurses, there were no differences between the four types of district nurses in the proportion of time spent with the various age and sex groups. They spent around two thirds of their patient time (excluding clinics) with female patients and much of it was with women aged 65 or more. Auxiliaries spent an even greater proportion of their time—almost three quarters—with women patients and in particular spent 49% of their time with women over 75, compared to 32% for district nurses.

Midwives spent three quarters of their time with women aged 16-44—those of child bearing age—and another 19% with babies less than one year old. They also spent very small amounts of time with male patients. People often do not or cannot distinguish between the different

Table 8.3 Time spent with patients in different types of clinic, by type of clinic

Type of clinic	Mid-wives	DN/ Midw.	HV	HV ass.	Schl. Nurse	Sch.N ass.	GP empl.	Fam. Plan.	Liai-son	Clinic
	%	%	%	%	%	%	%	%	%	%
Ante-natal and post-natal	73	49	7	1	*	–	3	1	–	1
Well baby, infant welfare, child health	1	–	54	25	8	9	1	*	8	15
Developmental assessment	1	1	11	5	2	–	*	–	1	3
Immunisation and vaccination	1	6	4	19	9	2	3	–	–	4
Mothercraft/parentcraft	8	8	3	–	*	–	–	–	–	–
Family planning	6	4	2	5	2	1	5	91	*	1
Well woman, cytology	3	1	1	7	2	3	3	1	–	2
Hearing and vision	–	*	5	16	16	6	–	–	–	4
School medicals/hygiene	*	–	2	7	45	52	1	*	8	7
Health education	1	–	2	–	1	–	–	*	–	–
GP surgery sessions	3	29	2	1	1	–	75	2	2	49
Other	3	2	7	14	14	27	9	4	70	14
Average hours spent on clinics (=100%)	*3.3*	*1.6*	*3.2*	*4.5*	*8.9*	*5.8*	*4.6*	*3.9*	*1.7*	*7.4*
Average number of patients seen per week in clinics	21	12	31	53	124	106	37	38	9	70
Average time per patient (minutes)	9	8	6	5	4	3	8	6	11	6
Number of nurses	313	91	967	63	409	35	252	202	48	48

Table 8.4 Time spent with patients (excluding that in clinics), by age and sex of patient, by type of nurse

Age and sex of patient	All DNs	DN SRN+	DN SRN−	DN SEN+	DN SEN−	Auxiliaries	Midwives
	%	%	%	%	%	%	%
Child up to one year	*	*	*	*	*	*	19
Child 1-4	*	*	1	*	*	*	1
Child 5-15	1	1	1	1	1	*	*
Woman 16-44	4	5	6	3	3	2	76
Woman 45-64	12	11	11	13	12	6	1
Woman 65-74	19	17	21	20	21	17	1
Woman 75-84	23	23	21	26	22	31	1
Woman 85+	9	10	8	8	9	18	*
(subtotals)	51 / 67	50 / 66	50 / 67	54 / 70	52 / 67	66 / 74	2 / 79
Man 16-44	2	3	2	2	1	1	*
Man 45-64	6	6	6	4	6	2	*
Man 65-74	11	11	11	9	11	7	*
Man 75-84	9	10	9	10	9	12	*
Man 85+	3	3	3	3	3	4	*
Groups	1	*	*	*	1	*	1
(subtotals)	23 / 31	24 / 33	23 / 31	23 / 28	24 / 31	* / 26	*
Average hours with patients, excluding clinics, (=100%)	15.7	15.6	12.4	18.8	17.1	14.8	13.6
Number of nurses	736	410	158	116	52	541	313

types of community nurses and it therefore seems quite appropriate to them to consult 'the nurse' about any health matter. This kind of situation accounts for the small amounts of time which nurses spent on age and sex groups which are not normally their responsibility. District nurse/midwives had a similar pattern to district nurses but spent a greater proportion of their time with younger women because of their midwifery function. Health visitors spent 62% of their time with children and only nine per cent with those aged 65 or more. Health visitor assistants, however, spent 29% of their time with children and a much greater proportion than health visitors, 57%, with those aged 65 or over.

As explained earlier, the types of nurses who spent most of their time on clinics and less than 10% of their time on home visits have been excluded from this table and from other tables relating to individual patient details. It is useful to note, however, that school nurses and assistants and family planning nurses tended to see one type of patient only—schoolchildren in the case of the first two and women of child bearing age (16–44) in the latter. GP employed practice nurses saw a wider spectrum of patients—for instance they spent a quarter of their time with female patients aged 16-44 and 60% of their time was spent with women patients. Another 10% was spent with children.

Turning to nurses with different patterns of working, Table 8.5 shows the proportions of time spent with patients in the five main age and sex groups by attached

and not attached nurses for district nurses, midwives, health visitors and auxiliaries. District nurses and auxiliaries who were not attached spent a greater proportion of time with men aged 65 and over than their attached counterparts—for auxiliaries the proportions were 30% and 18%. Attached district nurses and auxiliaries spent correspondingly higher proportions of their time with women aged 65 and over. There were no differences for midwives and health visitors.

Comparisons between nurses working with different numbers of practices were made for the same four types of nurses, as shown in Table 8.6. Here the district nurses and auxiliaries working with five or more practices (and the auxiliaries who had no GP contact) spent a greater proportion of their time with male patients aged 65 and over and a lower proportion with female patients of 65 and over, compared to those working with fewer practices. This ties in with the finding in the previous paragraph because in Chapter 5 we saw that the nurses working with five or more practices (and those who had no GP contact) were generally those who were not attached to general practice. There was no variation between midwives or health visitors working with different numbers of practices.

8.5 Proportion of time spent with different types of patients
Table 8.7 shows the proportion of time spent with different types of patients. District nurses spent 27% of their time with physically handicapped patients (which

Table 8.5 Time spent with patients by attached and not attached nurses: distribution by age and sex of patient

Age and sex of patient	District nurses Not attached	District nurses Attached	Midwives Not attached	Midwives Attached	Health visitors Not attached	Health visitors Attached	Auxiliaries Not attached	Auxiliaries Attached
	%	%	%	%	%	%	%	%
Child	1	1	19	19	63	69	*	*
Woman less than 65	14	16	78	78	22	18	8	8
Woman 65+	42	52	2	2	9	7	58	71
Man less than 65	12	8	*	*	2	2	4	3
Man 65+	31	23	1	1	3	4	30	18
Average hours with patients, excluding clinics, (=100%)	12.6	16.5	14.4	14.0	8.7	9.4	13.8	15.7
Number of nurses†	111	529	53	237	106	835	140	314

†Bases are smaller than on previous tables because full-time relief nurses have been excluded, as on previous tables relating to attachment.

DN/ Midw.	HV	HV ass.	Comm. Psych.	Geriatric	Liai-son	Clinic	Age and sex of patient
%	%	%	%	%	%	%	
3	36	9	*	*	5	1	Child up to 1 year
*	21	10	1	–	2	3	Child 1-4
1	5	10	5	*	5	5	Child 5-15
17	15	3	18	1	10	7	Woman 16-44
8	3	4	20	6	11	8	Woman 45-64
15	2	12	13	24	9	12	Woman 65-74
17	3	27	6	28	13	15	Woman 75-84
8	1	7	2	10	5	2	Woman 85+
40 { 65	6 { 24	46 { 53	21 { 59	62 { 69	29 { 48	29 { 44	(women subtotals)
2	1	*	12	*	9	5	Man 16-44
6	1	1	9	1	3	9	Man 45-64
10	1	4	5	12	9	18	Man 65-74
8	2	6	6	13	10	10	Man 75-84
4	*	1	*	4	3	*	Man 85+
22 { 30	3 { 5	11 { 12	7 { 28	29 { 30	22 { 34	28 { 42	(men subtotals)
1	9	6	7	1	6	5	Groups
15.0	9.3	6.1	12.3	12.2	8.1	4.8	Average hours with patients, excluding clinics, (=100%)
91	967	63	117	39	48	48	Number of nurses

Table 8.6 Time spent with patients by nurses working with different numbers of practices: distribution by age and sex of patient

Age and sex of patient	Number of practices†			
	1	2	3-4	5+
District nurses	%	%	%	%
Child	1	1	3	1
Woman less than 65	16	16	17	14
Woman 65+	54	53	52	36
Man less than 65	7	8	6	13
Man 65+	22	22	22	36
Average hours with patients excluding clinics, (=100%)	18.5	17.0	16.5	13.8
Number of nurses	288	126	90	108
Midwives	%	%	%	%
Child	18	21	17	15
Woman less than 65	76	79	75	84
Woman 65+	4	–	5	1
Man less than 65	*	*	1	*
Man 65+	2	–	2	*
Average hours with patients excluding clinics (=100%)	17.7	17.0	17.8	18.2
Number of nurses	53	74	72	81
Health visitors	%	%	%	%
Child	68	71	73	63
Woman less than 65	20	16	15	21
Woman 65+	7	7	7	9
Man less than 65	2	2	2	3
Man 65+	3	4	3	4
Average hours with patients excluding clinics (=100%)	12.8	12.5	12.3	12.5
Number of nurses	559	179	80	103
Auxiliaries	%	%	%	%
Child	*	*	*	*
Woman less than 65	7	9	9	8
Woman 65+	73	69	71	55
Man less than 65	2	3	2	5
Man 65+	18	19	18	32
Average hours with patients excluding clinics (=100%)	15.2	15.7	16.2	17.2
Number of nurses	160	85	75	48

†The small number of nurses who said they had no contact with GPs or did not know how many practices they worked with were excluded from the table.

included those with arthritis, rheumatism etc), 13% with elderly patients who did not have a specific condition and another 13% with patients with skin conditions such as sores and ulcers. There was little variation between the different types of district nurses although there was evidence of a tendency for the less qualified district nursing staff to spend a greater proportion of their time on elderly patients with no specific condition. Auxiliaries spent very little time with diabetics, skin condition patients or post-operative/hospital discharge patients compared with district nurses. They therefore spent higher proportions of time than district nurses with the groups they both saw most—the elderly and phsyically handicapped.

Midwives spent 90% of their time with expectant mothers and maternity cases. More than half of health visitors' time was spent with children and/or the person caring for them. Six per cent of their time included in the 'other' category was spent with problem families. Health visitor assistants spent higher proportions of their time than health visitors with the elderly and the physically handicapped—and less time with children.

Geriatric nurses also spent large proportions of their time with the elderly and physically handicapped. They spent another 13% of their time with the mentally ill (which included senile dementia and confusion) and 15% with cardio-vascular disease patients. Liaison nurses' time was fairly evenly distributed across all the different types of patients and clinic nurses spent almost half their time with chest disease patients.

GP employed practice nurses were excluded from the table because they spent only a small proportion of their time outside the practice. However the individual patients they did deal with were of a wide variety of types and contact had usually been initiated by the GP.

8.6 Proportion of time with patients by who initiated the contact

Table 8.8 shows the distribution of time spent with patients by who initiated the contact, for the different types of nurses. Looking first at district nurses there was some variation between the different types. Patient contacts which nurses had initiated themselves accounted for a third or more of the time of all types of district nurses but the SRNs with district training spent a greater proportion—45%—of their time on these. The SEN district nurses spent a larger proportion of their time on GP-initiated contacts and both SENs and SRNs without district training spent more time than other district nurses on contacts which had been initiated by other community nursing staff. Auxiliaries spent a particularly high proportion of time (38%) on the latter type of contacts compared to other types of staff.

Midwives spent over half of their time on patient contacts which they had initiated and hospitals were their other main source of referral (22%). Health visitors spent most of their time on contacts which they had initiated, apart from 12% spent on contacts initiated by the patient or their family. They also spent 10% of their time on birth notification visits to new born babies, which health visitor assistants did not do. The latter group spent 60% of their

time on self-initiated contacts and 10% on school-initiated contacts. Both spent only a small proportion of their time on GP-initiated contacts.

Community psychiatric nurses and liaison nurses spent around a quarter of their time on hospital-initiated contacts. The proportion of time spent on patient contacts initiated by other community nursing staff or other members of the practice team was very small for community psychiatric, liaison and clinic nurses and health visitors.

Considering the types of nurses who spent most of their time doing clinics, GP employed nurses' time was spent

Table 8.7 Time spent with patients (excluding that in clinics), by type of patient

Type of patient	All DNs	DN SRN+	DN SRN−	DN SEN+	DN SEN−	Auxil-iaries	Mid-wives	DN/ Midw.	HV	HV ass.	Comm. Psych.	Geria-tric	Liai-son	Clinic
	%	%	%	%	%	%	%	%	%	%	%	%	%	%
Expectant mother	*	*	*	*	*	*	22	3	4	1	*	−	*	*
Maternity	1	1	1	*	*	*	68	14	12	1	*	*	1	−
Child and person caring for it	1	1	1	*	*	*	5	1	53	10	*	*	5	4
Schoolchild and person caring for it	*	1	*	*	1	*	*	*	4	12	1	−	1	5
Post-op/hosp. discharge	7	8	7	5	6	*	1	5	1	2	*	3	4	4
Terminal/deteriorating	9	10	9	9	9	5	1	7	1	2	*	5	2	2
Physical handicap	27	26	24	31	25	41	1	19	1	15	*	27	11	11
Mental handicap	*	*	1	*	1	1	−	*	1	3	9	1	3	−
Mental illness	4	4	3	4	4	5	*	2	4	10	80	13	17	3
Chest disease	3	3	3	3	3	2	*	2	1	3	*	6	12	48
Cardio-vascular disease	11	12	12	9	9	17	*	11	1	8	*	15	13	3
Skin inc. sores and ulcers	13	12	14	14	13	1	1	13	*	1	−	3	1	3
Diabetic	7	7	7	8	7	1	*	5	1	1	*	3	5	2
Elderly-non specific	13	11	13	14	20	25	1	14	5	25	2	22	10	5
Other	4	4	5	3	2	2	*	4	9	6	8	2	15	10
Average hours with patients, excluding clinics, (=100%)	15.7	15.6	12.4	18.8	17.1	14.8	13.6	15.0	9.3	6.1	12.3	12.2	8.1	4.8
Number of nurses	736	410	158	116	52	541	313	91	967	63	117	39	48	48

Table 8.8 Time spent with patients (excluding that in clinics), by who initiated the contact

Who initiated contact	All DNs	DN SRN+	DN SRN−	DN SEN+	DN SEN−	Auxil-iaries	Mid-wives	DN/ Midw.	HV	HV ass.	Comm. psych	Geria-tric	Liai-son	Clinic
	%	%	%	%	%	%	%	%	%	%	%	%	%	%
Birth notification†	*	*	*	−	−	−	4	2	10	*	−	−	1	2
The nurse—first visit	1	1	1	*	*	1	5	1	5	6	2	7	4	2
The nurse—routine/follow-up	40	45	35	34	32	41	50	35	58	53	51	36	35	33
Patient or their family	1	1	1	1	1	1	4	1	12	5	3	11	9	3
GP	33	30	33	38	40	8	3	37	6	10	6	17	18	36
Other member of practice team	3	2	3	5	5	10	2	1	1	5	3	3	6	7
Other community nursing staff	10	8	16	8	15	38	9	7	1	4	3	9	1	*
Hospital	12	12	11	14	6	1	22	15	3	4	28	14	24	12
School	*	−	−	*	*	*	*	−	1	10	*	−	*	2
Other	*	1	*	*	1	*	1	1	3	3	4	3	2	3
Average hours with patients, excluding clinics, (=100%)	15.7	15.6	12.4	18.8	17.1	14.8	13.6	15.0	9.3	6.1	12.3	12.2	8.1	4.8
Number of nurses	736	410	158	116	52	541	313	91	967	63	117	39	48	48

†Described as 'primary visit to new born baby' on list of codes

Table 8.9 Time spent with patients by attached and not attached nurses: distribution by who initiated contact

Who initiated contact	District nurses		Midwives		Health visitors		Auxiliaries	
	Not attached	Attached	Not attached	Attached	Not attached	Attached	Not attached	Attached
	%	%	%	%	%	%	%	%
Birth notification†	*	*	4	4	9	10	−	−
The nurse—first visit	1	*	4	6	4	5	*	*
The nurse— routine/follow-up	41	41	48	50	53	58	25	49
Patient or their family	1	1	4	4	14	12	*	*
GP	24	35	1	4	3	7	6	9
Other member of practice team	3	3	2	2	1	1	8	11
Other community nursing staff	18	7	10	8	2	1	59	31
Hospital	11	12	27	21	8	2	2	*
School	*	*	−	*	3	1	*	−
Other	1	1	*	1	3	3	*	*
Average hours with patients, excluding clinics, (=100%)	12.6	16.5	14.4	14.0	8.7	9.4	13.8	15.7
Number of nurses	111	529	53	237	106	835	140	314

†Described as 'primary visit to new born baby' on list of codes

mainly on GP-initiated contacts and school nurses and assistants spent most of their non-clinic time on contacts initiated by themselves or by schools.

Table 8.9 shows the proportions of time which attached and not attached nurses spent with patients by who initiated the patient contact. There were no significant differences for midwives and health visitors. Looking at district nurses and auxiliaries, the proportion of time spent with patients when other community nursing staff had initiated the contact was higher for the nurses who were not attached than for those who were. Attached district nurses spent a higher proportion of time on patient contacts initiated by the GP than the not attached—this may indicate that attached district nurses *do* work in closer contact with GPs. Attached auxiliaries spent more time—49%—on routine or follow-up contacts which they initiated themselves than the not attached who spent only 25% of their time on this. This may indicate that attached auxiliaries are given responsibility for some routine and follow-up visits, particularly as the not attached auxiliaries spent correspondingly more time on visits initiated by other community nursing staff.

Table 8.10 shows the proportions of time which nurses working with different numbers of practices spent with patients by who initiated the contact. Again there were no differences for midwives and health visitors. District nurses who worked with five or more practices had the same pattern as not attached district nurses—they spent a lower proportion of time on GP initiated patient contacts than district nurses working with fewer practices and a higher proportion of time on contacts initiated by other community nursing staff. Similarly auxiliaries working with five or more practices and those who had no GP contact spent a greater proportion of time on contacts initiated by other community nursing staff, like the not attached auxiliaries.

Table 8.10 Time spent with patients by nurses working with different numbers of practices: distribution by who initiated contact

Who initiated contact	Number of practices†			
	1	2	3-4	5+
District nurses	%	%	%	%
Birth notification††	*	*	*	*
The nurse—first visit	1	*	1	1
The nurse—routine/follow-up	43	36	45	42
Patient or their family	1	1	1	2
GP	36	38	33	22
Other member of practice team	3	4	3	5
Other community nursing staff	6	6	6	15
Hospital	10	14	10	12
School	–	*	–	*
Other	1	1	1	1
Average hours with patients, excluding clinics (=100%)	18.5	17.0	16.5	13.8
Number of nurses	288	126	90	108
Midwives	%	%	%	%
Birth notification††	5	5	2	3
The nurse—first visit	5	6	5	5
The nurse—routine/follow-up	43	50	55	49
Patient or their family	5	4	3	5
GP	7	3	4	2
Other member of practice team	3	1	2	2
Other community nursing staff	7	10	7	9
Hospital	25	21	22	23
School	*	*	–	–
Other	*	*	*	2
Average hours with patients, excluding clinics (=100%)	17.7	17.0	17.8	18.2
Number of nurses	53	74	72	81
Health visitors	%	%	%	%
Birth notification††	9	10	9	10
The nurse—first visit	6	6	5	4
The nurse—routine/follow-up	58	57	59	57
Patient or their family	13	11	10	12
GP	6	7	7	3
Other member of practice team	1	1	1	1
Other community nursing staff	1	1	2	1
Hospital	2	2	2	7
School	1	2	2	1
Other	3	3	3	4
Average hours with patients, excluding clinics (=100%)	12.8	12.5	12.3	12.5
Number of nurses	559	179	80	103
Auxiliaries	%	%	%	%
Birth notification††	–	–	–	–
The nurse—first visit	*	1	*	*
The nurse—routine/follow-up	46	43	51	45
Patient or their family	*	1	*	*
GP	11	9	9	4
Other member of practice team	13	9	8	4
Other community nursing staff	29	37	32	47
Hospital	1	*	*	–
School	–	*	*	–
Other	*	*	*	–
Average hours with patients, excluding clinics (=100%)	15.2	15.7	16.2	17.2
Number of nurses	160	85	75	48

†The small number of nurses who said they had no contact with GPs or did not know how many practices they worked with were excluded from the table.

††Described as 'primary visit to new born baby' in list of codes.

51

Appendix to Chapter 8

In Sections 8.4 and 8.5 we looked at the proportions of time which the various types of nurses spent with patients of different types and different age and sex groups. It is possible to carry such analysis further by looking at each of the five major age and sex groups (children, women aged less than 65, women of 65 and over, men aged less than 65 and men of 65 and over) and breaking down the time spent with different types of patients within each group of the various types of nurses. This is done in Tables A8.1 to A8.4.† Types of nurses who only spent a very small amount or proportion of time with a particular age and sex group have been excluded from the table relating to that group.

The tables can be used in several different ways. An examination of Tables A8.1 and A8.2, for instance, compares the proportions of time spent with different types of women patients aged less than 65 with those aged 65 or more. Tables A8.3 and A8.4 can be used to make a similar comparison for men. Alternatively comparing Table A8.1 with A8.3, or Table A8.2 with A8.4, shows differences between the sexes for patients in the same age group. The variation between different types of nurses can be examined as well as the variation between the four different age and sex groups for the same type of nurse.

For example, consider Tables A8.2 and A8.4 to look at the differences between elderly female patients and elderly male patients. Looking first at district nurses they spent larger proportions of their time with the elderly men with those who had chest disease, cardio-vascular disease or a terminal/deteriorating condition. The physically handicapped accounted for the largest single proportion of time for both sexes. Clinic nurses spent 56% of their time with elderly men or those with chest disease but spent so little time with elderly women that they did not even appear on the table. These findings are what might be expected from our knowledge of the different illnesses and causes of death which apply to the different sexes.

Since different readers will be interested in patients of different ages, types etc and since there are so many possible comparisons and combinations we have not attempted to comment on the many variations. We provide the tables and hope that individual readers will look closely at the comparisons of interest to them.

†Time spent with children has not been broken down in this way as a large proportion of children visited were of the type "child and person caring for it".

Table A8.1 Time spent with female patients 16-64 (excluding clinics), by type of patient

Type of patient	All DNs	DN SRN+	DN SRN−	DN SEN+	DN SEN−	Auxil-iaries	Mid-wives	DN/ Midw.	HV	Comm. Psych.	Liaison
	%	%	%	%	%	%	%	%	%	%	%
Expectant mother	1	1	2	*	*	*	27	13	16	*	1
Maternity	3	4	5	1	*	*	69	43	10	1	−
Woman caring for child	1	1	1	1	3	1	2	1	38	2	1
Post-operative/hospital discharge	14	15	15	13	10	1	1	6	2	−	6
Terminal/deteriorating	15	16	10	16	10	10	*	7	1	*	*
Physical handicap	35	34	30	40	42	64	1	12	4	1	6
Mental handicap/illness	3	3	5	4	6	4	*	1	18	92†	31
Chest disease	2	2	2	2	1	1	*	2	1	*	9
Cardio-vascular disease	4	4	5	3	4	11	*	5	1	*	8
Skin including sores and ulcers	9	8	10	9	10	1	*	4	*	−	*
Diabetic	6	6	5	6	8	1	*	2	2	*	6
Other	7	6	10	5	6	6	*	4	7	4	32
Average hours with female patients 16-64 (=100%)	*2.3*	*2.3*	*1.9*	*2.9*	*2.5*	*1.1*	*8.4*	*3.5*	*1.3*	*3.8*	*1.1*
Number of nurses	736	410	158	116	52	541	313	91	967	117	48

†Consists of 86% mental illness, 6% mental handicap

Table A8.2 Time spent with female patients aged 65+ (excluding clinics), by type of patient

Type of patient	All DNs	DN SRN+	DN SRN−	DN SEN+	DN SEN−	Auxil-iaries	DN/ Midw.	HV ass.	Comm. Psych	Geria-tric	Liaison
	%	%	%	%	%	%	%	%	%	%	%
Post-operative/hospital discharge	3	4	4	2	2	*	3	1	*	3	5
Terminal/deteriorating	7	7	7	6	7	3	5	2	−	5	2
Physical handicap	25	24	22	29	23	41	21	24	−	29	19
Mental handicap/illness	5	5	4	5	5	6	4	15	93†	15	6
Chest disease	2	2	2	2	2	2	1	3	−	4	3
Cardio-vascular disease	12	13	12	10	9	15	14	11	*	15	10
Skin including sores and ulcers	16	16	17	15	16	1	16	1	−	4	4
Diabetic	9	9	8	9	9	1	7	1	−	3	6
Elderly-non specific	18	16	20	20	26	30	24	40	5	21	25
Other	3	4	4	2	1	1	5	2	2	1	20
Average hours spent with female patients 65+ (= 100%)	*7.3*	*7.1*	*5.7*	*9.7*	*8.7*	*9.0*	*5.6*	*1.8*	*2.2*	*6.7*	*1.5*
Number of patients	736	410	158	116	52	541	91	63	117	39	48

†The entire 93% referred to mental illness—no time was spent with mentally handicapped women aged 65+

Table A8.3 Time spent with male patients aged 16-64 (excluding clinics), by type of patient

Type of patient	All DNs	DN SRN+	DN SRN-	DN SEN+	DN SEN-	Auxil- iaries	DN/ Midw.	Comm. Psych.	Liaison
	%	%	%	%	%	%	%	%	%
Post-operative/hospital discharge	20	21	18	15	28	–	19	–	4
Terminal/deteriorating	10	11	13	7	8	13	19	–	5
Physical handicap	35	35	34	42	25	60	27	–	6
Mental handicap/illness	4	1	4	1	3	6	2	92†	56††
Chest disease	3	6	3	2	1	3	1	–	10
Cardio-vascular disease	6	6	6	6	7	15	9	–	1
Skin including sores and ulcers	8	6	5	13	14	1	10	–	2
Diabetic	6	5	9	7	5	–	5	–	2
Other	8	9	8	7	9	2	8	8	15
Average hours spent with male patients 16-64 (=100%)	*1.2*	*1.2*	*1.0*	*1.1*	*1.2*	*0.4*	*1.1*	*2.2*	*0.7*
Number of nurses	736	410	158	116	52	541	91	117	48

†Consists of 9% mental handicap and 83% mental illness
††Consists of 1% mental handicap and 55% mental illness

Table A8.4 Time spent with male patients 65+ (excluding clinics), by type of patient

Type of patient	All DNs	DN SRN+	DN SRN-	DN SEN+	DN SEN-	Auxil- iaries	DN/ Midw.	Comm. Psych.	Geria- tric	Liaison	Clinic
	%	%	%	%	%	%	%	%	%	%	%
Post-operative/hospital discharge	5	6	5	3	5	*	4	–	2	4	4
Terminal/deteriorating	12	13	11	10	14	10	10	1	4	1	2
Physical handicap	21	21	21	24	16	29	16	–	19	12	13
Mental handicap/illness	4	4	4	3	4	3	2	91†	12	8	5
Chest disease	6	6	6	5	7	6	4	–	11	18	56
Cardio-vascular disease	17	19	18	14	13	28	18	–	18	31	6
Skin including sores and ulcers	11	9	14	15	12	1	19	–	1	1	2
Diabetic	6	6	6	8	6	1	6	–	2	5	–
Elderly—non specific	14	13	12	15	21	21	18	6	27	13	2
Other	4	3	3	3	2	1	3	2	4	7	10
Average hours spent with male patients 65+ (= 100%)	*3.4*	*3.5*	*2.6*	*4.0*	*4.0*	*3.0*	*3.0*	*0.8*	*3.2*	*1.2*	*0.6*
Number of nurses	736	410	158	116	52	541	91	117	39	48	48

†Consists of 1% mental handicap and 90% mental illness

9 Detailed examination of activities with patients/clients

In Chapters 6 and 7 we looked at the working time recorded in the diaries by the different types of nurses working in the community and at the proportion of that time which was spent on travelling. In this chapter the time spent on travelling is excluded and we examine firstly 'activity time' and then, for the rest of the chapter, time spent with patients.

'Activity time' as explained in Chapter 6, is the term used to refer to total working time excluding travel time ie time spent on non-clinical activities and activities with patients (including unspecified activities). Table 9.1 looks at the proportions of time spent on the activities which make up the total activity time. It is now clear that more than half of activity time is spent on non-clinical activities by health visitor assistants, GP employed practice nurses, community psychiatric and liaison nurses. These are things such as telephone calls, meetings, clerical and administrative tasks etc.

The time spent on the various non-clinical activities is looked at in detail in Chapter 10 so for the rest of this chapter we shall also exclude time spent on non-clinical activities and focus solely on time spent with patients. All subsequent tables therefore have time with patients—not activity time—as their base.

9.1 Proportion of time with patients spent on the four main areas of activity

The 22 categories used in the diary to record activities with patients are listed below.

ACTIVITIES WITH PATIENTS/CLIENTS

Technical tests, assessments, screening and surveillance

10 Scalp inspection
   Vision testing
   Audiometry, hearing test
   Cervical smear
   Taking swabs, blood/urine/faeces sample
   Blood pressure
   Pregnancy, skin testing
   Weight, height, temperature, pulse, respiration
11 ECG
   Breast palpation, examination
   Ante or post-natal examination
   Child development, observation
   Health surveillance

Technical procedures

12 Injection, vaccination, immunisation
   Eye/ear treatments, syringing

13 Inserting/removing stitches, plaster of paris, cervical collar
   Dressings, care of pressure sores
   Enema, rectal suppository, washout, manual removal
   Vaginal suppository, pessary, douche
   Catheterisation, bladder washout
   Stoma care
   Rehabilitation exercises
14 Home/GP unit delivery, attending minor ops

Other nursing care

15 Routine nursing care, bathing, prevention of incontinence/pressure sores
16 Other personal care:
   Help with lavatory, commode, bed pan
   Help with washing, dressing, nappy changing
   Care for hair, nails, feet
   Feed or give medicine

17 Home help type care:
   Prepare food and drinks
   Housework, washing clothes, dishes etc
   Shopping, collecting pension, benefits, prescriptions
18 Supervision of patient/client
19 Assessment visits for home conditions/social/needs for equipment etc
   Delivering and instructing in use of aids/equipment
20 Other clinical (specify)

Advice, counselling, reassurance, education

21 Pregnancy, labour, family planning, vasectomy, sterilisation, abortion
22 Diet, nutrition, infant feeding, immunisation, vaccination
23 Parentcraft/children—development, management, abuse, adoption, fostering
24 Personal, emotional, social problems eg marital, bereavement, housing, financial
25 Physical health problems
26 Mental health problems inc. addiction, alcoholism, depression
27 Health education—general
28 Advice to relatives—nursing care etc.
29 Reassurance—general
30 Social—chatting and listening
31 Other (specify)

The examples given for each category provide an indication of the kinds of activities included in each category but are not an exhaustive list. Nurses used the examples as a guide when selecting the appropriate code for an activity which was not specifically listed. As explained in Chapter 6, time spent on unspecified activities has been included in the totals of time spent with patients and is usually shown as a separate category on the tables.

In Table 9.2 activities with patients are divided into four broad categories—technical tests, assessments, screening and surveillance (codes 10 and 11 on the diary), technical procedures (codes 12, 13 and 14), other nursing care (codes 15 to 20) and advice, counselling, reassurance and education (codes 21-30). There was much variation in the proportion of time with patients spent on these four areas of activity by the different types of nurses.

District nurses spent about two fifths of this time on technical procedures and about another two fifths on other nursing care. There was little variation between the district nurses. The SENs tended to spend a higher proportion of time than the SRNs on other nursing care but the difference was small. Auxiliaries spent most (84%) of their time with patients on other nursing care activities.

Midwives had a different pattern—they spent two fifths of their 'with patients' time on technical tests, another third on advice and only small proportions on technical procedures and other nursing care. Joint duty district nurse/midwives had a pattern of work which was more similar to that of district nurses.

Health visitors spent 73% of their time with patients providing advice and counselling and only small proportions of time on the other activities.

School nurses and assistants spent more than half their time on technical tests, assessment etc. Family planning nurses spent 46% of their time with patients giving advice and just over a third of their time on technical tests. Clinic nurses also spent just over a third of their time on technical tests but spent a similar proportion of their time on technical procedures. Community psychiatric geriatric and liaison nurses both spent more than half of their time with patients on advisory activities and geriatric nurses spent a third of their time on other nursing care.

There was little variation in the proportion of time spent by attached and not attached nurses on these four categories of activities with patients. Comparisons between attached and not attached district nurses, midwives, health visitors and auxiliaries were made and are shown in Table 9.3. There were no differences between nurses working with different numbers of practices.

9.2 Proportion of time with patients spent on each activity

Table 9.4 gives a more detailed breakdown of the time spent with patients. Again there was much variation between the different types of nurses.

We saw in Table 9.2 that *district nurses* spent large proportions of their time on technical procedures and other nursing care. Table 9.4 shows that the 40% of time spent carrying out technical procedures included 11% for injections and 28% for other procedures such as changing dressings and inserting and removing stitches. The 38% spent on other nursing care included 23% on routine nursing care and 8% on other personal care. There was little variation between the district nurses except that SENs without a district nursing qualification spent a

Table 9.1 Proportions of activity time spent on various activities, by type of nurse

Type of activity	All DNs	DN SRN+	DN SRN−	DN SEN+	DN SEN−	Auxil- iaries	GP empl.	Mid- wives	DN/ Midw.	HV	HV ass.	Schl. Nurse	Sch.N ass.	Fam. Plan.	Comm. Psych.	Geria- tric	Liai son	Clinic
	%	%	%	%	%	%	%	%	%	%	%	%	%	%	%	%	%	%
Non-clinical	35	37	35	32	28	20	58	37	39	55	53	48	47	42	52	49	67	48
With patients:																		
technical tests, assessments, screening and surveillance	1	2	2	1	1	2	13	25	8	6	14	28	35	20	*	1	1	18
technical procedures	26	25	25	28	27	3	19	5	19	1	6	6	3	2	4	4	5	17
other nursing care	25	23	24	27	34	67	2	8	18	1	4	5	9	7	5	16	5	6
advice, counselling, reassurance, education	11	11	12	10	9	6	7	20	12	33	18	10	3	27	37	26	21	8
Unspecified	2	2	2	2	1	2	1	5	4	4	5	3	3	2	2	4	1	3
Average activity hours (= 100%)	*25.5*	*26.8*	*20.2*	*28.4*	*24.0*	*19.4*	*18.4*	*26.9*	*27.2*	*27.5*	*22.4*	*25.9*	*28.4*	*9.8*	*28.1*	*24.5*	*29.8*	*23.2*
Number of nurses	736	410	158	116	52	541	252	313	91	967	63	409	35	202	117	39	48	48

Table 9.2 Proportion of time with patients spent on different activities, by type of nurse

Activities with patients	All DNs	DN SRN+	DN SRN−	DN SEN+	DN SEN−	Auxil- iaries	GP empl.	Mid- wives	DN/ Midw.	HV	HV ass.	Schl. Nurse	Sch.N ass.	Fam. Plan.	Comm. Psych.	Geria- tric	Liai son	Clinic
	%	%	%	%	%	%	%	%	%	%	%	%	%	%	%	%	%	%
Technical tests, assessments, screening and surveillance	2	3	4	1	2	3	30	40	13	14	30	53	66	34	1	2	2	35
Technical procedures	40	39	38	42	39	4	47	7	32	2	12	12	6	4	7	7	14	33
Other nursing care	38	37	37	40	44	84	5	13	29	3	9	10	16	12	11	32	15	11
Advice, counselling, reassurance, education	17	17	17	15	13	7	16	32	19	73	38	19	7	46	76	51	64	16
Unspecified	3	4	4	2	2	2	2	8	7	8	11	6	5	4	5	8	5	5
Average hours on activities with patients (= 100%)	*16.6*	*16.9*	*13.2*	*19.3*	*17.4*	*15.4*	*7.7*	*16.9*	*16.6*	*12.5*	*10.6*	*13.5*	*15.0*	*5.6*	*13.4*	*12.6*	*9.8*	*12.2*
Number of nurses	736	410	158	116	52	541	252	313	91	967	63	409	35	202	117	39	48	48

slightly higher proportion of time than other district nurses on routine nursing care. The SRNs spent a slightly higher proportion of their time than the SENs on advisory activities but the difference was small.

Auxiliaries spent a much greater proportion of their time than district nurses on routine nursing care and other personal care and eight per cent on supervision of patients—these three categories accounted for more than four fifths of their time with patients. However they did not, as one might have expected, spend a larger proportion of time than district nurses on home help type care.

Since little information is available about the activities on which *GP employed practice nurses* are engaged it is worth noting that a quarter of their time with patients was spent on technical tests, another quarter giving injections, 20% on other technical procedures and 16% on advisory activities. Only five per cent of their time was spent on the routine and other nursing care activities.

Midwives had a different pattern to district nurses. Table 9.2 showed that they spent two fifths of their time

carrying out technical tests, assessments, screening and surveillance. Table 9.4 shows that 13% was spent on technical tests and 27% on technical examinations and surveillance. They spent one third of their time on advisory activities and five per cent on deliveries and minor operations.

Health visitors had a different pattern again and spent 73% of their time with clients on advisory activities. *Health visitor assistants* spent a much smaller proportion of their time providing advice—37%—and did technical tests for 27% of their time. *School nurses and assistants* spent large proportions of their time with patients doing technical tests—46% and 65% respectively. School nurses spent a higher proportion of their time than the assistants on advisory activities.

Technical tests accounted for 31% of the 34% of time that *family planning nurses* spent carrying out technical tests, assessments, screening and surveillance. They also spent almost half of their time on advisory activities. *Community psychiatric and liaison nurses* spent much of their time—76% and 64% respectively—providing advice. *Geriatric nurses* spent a much greater proportion of time

Table 9.3 Proportion of time with patients spent on different activities, by attachment

Activities with patients	District nurses		Midwives		Health visitors		Auxiliaries	
	Not attached	Attached	Not attached	Attached	Not attached	Attached	Not attached	Attached
	%	%	%	%	%	%	%	%
Technical tests, assessments, screening and surveillance	2	3	35	41	11	14	7	1
Technical procedures	36	40	9	7	2	2	2	3
Other nursing care	44	37	19	11	5	3	82	89
Advice, counselling, reassurance, education	16	17	31	32	73	73	8	5
Unspecified	2	3	6	9	9	8	1	2
Average hours spent on activities with patients (= 100%)	*12.9*	*17.6*	*17.0*	*17.5*	*11.7*	*12.7*	*15.0*	*15.8*
Number of nurses	111	529	53	237	106	835	140	314

Table 9.4 Proportion of time with patients spent on each type of clinical activity†, by type of nurse

Type of activity	All DNs	DN SRN+	DN SRN−	DN SEN+	DN SEN−	Auxil- iaries	GP empl.	Mid- wives	DN/ Midw.	HV	HV ass.	Schl. Nurse	Sch.N ass.	Fam. Plan.	Comm. Psych.	Geria- tric	Liai- son	Clinic
	%	%	%	%	%	%	%	%	%	%	%	%	%	%	%	%	%	%
Technical tests, assessments, screening and surveillance:																		
technical tests	2	2	2	1	1	3	24	13	4	6	27	46	65	31	*	2	2	25
technical examinations	*	1	2	*	1	*	7	27	9	8	3	7	2	3	*	*	*	10
Technical procedures:																		
injections etc††	11	11	10	11	10	1	25	*	8	1	11	8	2	1	6	2	3	17
other technical procedures†††	28	27	27	30	28	3	20	2	23	*	*	3	2	1	1	5	9	15
delivery, minor op	1	1	1	1	1	*	2	5	1	1	1	1	1	2	1	*	2	1
Other nursing care:																		
routine nursing care	23	22	22	24	29	49	1	4	17	*	−	1	2	1	*	9	3	1
other personal care	8	8	9	10	10	24	*	3	6	*	*	2	7	*	*	6	1	1
home help type care	2	2	1	2	1	2	*	*	1	*	*	*	1	*	2	2	*	*
supervision of patient	2	2	2	2	3	8	*	1	2	1	2	1	2	3	3	2	2	6
assessment visits	2	2	2	2	1	1	*	3	2	1	4	1	*	1	3	13	6	1
other clinical	1	1	1	*	*	*	3	2	1	1	3	5	4	7	3	*	3	2
Advice, counselling, reassurance and education	17	17	17	15	13	7	16	32	19	73	38	19	7	46	76	51	64	16
Unspecified	3	4	4	2	2	2	2	8	7	8	11	6	5	4	5	8	5	5
Average hours spent on activities with patients (= 100%)	*16.6*	*16.9*	*13.2*	*19.3*	*17.8*	*15.4*	*7.7*	*16.9*	*16.6*	*12.5*	*10.6*	*13.5*	*15.0*	*5.6*	*13.4*	*12.6*	*9.8*	*12.2*
Number of nurses	736	410	158	116	52	541	252	313	91	967	63	409	35	202	117	39	48	48

†For full description of each activity, see list of codes
††Includes injection, vaccination, immunisation, eye/ear treatments, syringing
†††Includes inserting/removing stitches, dressings, enema—see code 13 for full list of examples

than district nurses on advisory activities and assessment visits and a lower proportion on technical procedures and nursing care. *Clinic nurses* had a pattern of activities that was most like that of GP employed practice nurses.

When different patterns of working were compared, there were no significant differences, between attached and not attached district nurses, midwives and health visitors, in the proportions of time spent on the various individual activities. There were some differences, however, for auxiliaries. When only the four broad activity areas were examined in Table 9.3 the difference between not attached and attached auxiliaries in the proportion of time spent on other nursing care was not significant (82% and 89%). Looking at the individual activities, however, auxiliaries who were not attached spent a greater proportion of their time than the attached on supervision of patients—17% compared to 1%. Attached auxiliaries spent a correspondingly higher proportion of time on routine nursing care.

There were no differences between nurses working with different numbers of practices.

9.3 Advice, counselling, reassurance and education

A more detailed breakdown of advisory activities is given in Table 9.5 which shows the time spent on the different types of advice and reassurance as a proportion of the time spent on all advisory activities. Health visitors, community psychiatric nurses, geriatric and liaison nurses spent the most time—six hours on average—on advisory activities and they are also the types of nurses who spent more than half of their time with patients on advisory activities.

District nurses spent most of their time on general reassurance and on the category described as 'social—chatting and listening' which will be referred to as 'social conversation'. The SENs spent a higher proportion of time on social conversation than the SRNs. All types of district nurses spent a greater proportion of time on advice to relatives than did other kinds of nurses. *Auxiliaries* spent a particularly high proportion of time—49%—on social conversation. Much of the reassurance and social conversation carried out by district nurses and auxiliaries was done at the same time as another clinical activity such as giving an injection or routine nursing

care. One of the guidelines for completion of the diary explained that nurses who carried out two activities at the same time—such as chatting whilst bathing a patient—should divide the time as accurately as possible between the two activities.

Generally the different types of nurses spent large proportions of time on the areas of advice relevant to their particular job, as one would expect. *Midwives* for example, gave advice chiefly on diet/infant feeding/immunisation (28%) followed by pregnancy/labour/family planning (19%) and parentcraft (13%). *Health visitor assistants* spent greater proportions of time on reassurance and chatting than health visitors and there was a similar variation between school nurse assistants and school nurses. *School nurses* spent the highest proportions of time of all the nurses on physical health problems and health education. *Community psychiatric and geriatric nurses* and health visitor assistants spent the highest proportions of time advising on personal problems—15% and 19%.

We saw in Chapter 7 that there was little variation in the proportion of working time spent on advisory activities between attached and not attached nurses or between nurses working with different numbers of practices. Not surprisingly, therefore, there was no variation in the proportion of time spent on the different kinds of advice between attached and not attached nurses or between nurses working with different numbers of practices.

9.4 Proportion of activities carried out during clinics and home visits

Table 9.6 looks at the time spent on each of the four main areas of activity with patients—technical tests, technical procedures, other nursing care and advice—and, for each area of activity, shows how the time spent on this activity is proportioned between clinics, home visits and other patient contacts. (These three types of contact with patients were discussed in Chapter 8.) Proportions have not been calculated when nurses spent only half an hour or less on a particular area of activity.

The table can be used in two different ways. Firstly each part of the table focuses on one of the four areas of activity and therefore shows the variation between the different types of nurses in the proportion of time relating

Table 9.5 Proportion of time spent on the different advisory activities, by type of nurse

Type of advice	All DNs	DN SRN+	DN SRN-	DN SEN+	DN SEN-	Auxil- iaries	GP empl.	Mid- wives	DN/ Midw.	HV	HV ass.	Schl. Nurse	Sch.N ass.	Fam. Plan.	Comm. Psych.	Geri- tric	Liai- son	Clinic
	%	%	%	%	%	%	%	%	%	%	%	%	%	%	%	%	%	%
Pregnancy, family planning etc.	*	1	1	*	1	1	21	19	8	5	2	7	–	72	*	–	1	6
Diet, infant feeding, vaccination	3	3	3	1	1	1	11	28	14	26	15	5	–	2	1	6	3	6
Parentcraft/children	*	*	1	–	2	–	1	13	9	21	1	4	1	*	2	*	2	1
Personal problems	10	10	10	9	6	3	11	5	8	12	15	6	2	6	15	19	9	10
Physical health problems	7	8	5	4	4	2	10	1	3	7	12	24	7	1	2	16	8	14
Mental health problems	2	2	2	2	5	1	2	*	1	3	3	1	–	1	35	7	11	2
Health education (general)	3	4	3	3	2	*	2	2	4	3	7	6	14	2	3	2	5	1	5
To relatives	17	18	14	15	17	9	5	2	12	2	3	4	5	*	10	5	9	11
Reassurance—general	30	29	32	35	28	22	12	15	21	7	21	10	17	6	12	19	16	20
Social—chatting & listening	27	24	28	31	34	49	12	11	20	7	17	17	28	6	15	22	10	21
Other	1	1	1	*	*	12	13	2	1	3	5	8	38	3	6	1	30	4
Average hours spent on advisory activities (= 100%)	2.8	2.9	2.3	2.8	2.3	1.1	1.2	5.5	3.2	9.1	4.1	2.5	1.0	2.6	10.3	6.4	6.2	2.0
Number of nurses	736	410	158	116	52	541	252	313	91	967	63	409	35	202	117	39	48	48

to that area of activity spent on clinics, home visits and other contacts. For example part (i), which relates to technical tests and assessments, shows that only a quarter of the time that midwives and district nurse/midwives devoted to technical tests and assessments was spent in clinics and over 70% was spent on home visits. Health visitors' time was more evenly divided between clinics and home visits whereas the majority of family planning and GP employed nurses' time was spent in clinics.

It is important to remember that the percentages are based on the time spent on a particular area of activity and not on the total time spent with patients. Part (iii) of the table, for instance—other nursing care—shows that liaison nurses spent a high proportion of that time—85%—on home visits. But this does not mean that liaison nurses spent most of their time on home visits because the 85% is based on the relatively small amount of time—1.4 hours—spent on other nursing care. We can see in part (iv) that liaison nurses spent much more of their time on advisory activities—6.2 hours—and this was more evenly distributed between home visits and other types of contact.

The second way of using the table is to take a particular type of nurse and look at the variation between the four areas of activity in the proportions of time spent on clinics, home visits and other contacts. For example Table 8.1 showed that, overall, health visitors spent 26% of their time with patients in clinics and 56% on home visits. Table 9.6 shows that a large proportion of their time on technical tests and assessments—50%—was in clinics whereas the majority of their time on advisory activities—68%—was spent in clients' homes during home visits. They spent very little time on the other two areas of activity.

It is interesting to consider the data in another way. Instead of focussing on each area of activity and dividing the time between clinics, home visits etc we can focus on the time spent on clinics or home visits and proportion that time between the different areas of activity. Sections 9.5 and 9.6 examine the data in this way.

9.5 Clinics

Table 9.2 showed the proportions of all time with patients spent on the four main areas of activity. Table 9.7 provides corresponding information for the time spent on clinics only. As in previous chapters nurses who spent only a small proportion of time on clinics have been excluded from the table.

Midwives spent half of their time in clinics doing technical tests and assessments and another third giving advice. Most of their clinic work was in ante-natal and post-natal clinics. Joint duty district nurse/midwives had the same pattern in their ante and post-natal clinics but they also did GP surgery sessions and in these spent a greater proportion of time on technical procedures—this is reflected in the overall proportions shown in the table.

Health visitors spent the greatest proportion of clinic time amongst the different types of nurses—60%—on advice. This was mainly in clinics connected with young children—well baby, infant welfare, child health and developmental assessment clinics. *Health visitor assistants* also did these kinds of clinics but spent a much smaller proportion of time than health visitors on advice

Table 9.6 Proportion of time spent on clinics and home visits for the four main areas of activity with patients, by type of nurse

Type of contact with patient	All DNs	DN SRN+	DN SRN−	DN SEN+	DN SEN−	Auxiliaries	GP empl.	Midwives	DN/ Midw.	HV	HV ass.	Schl. Nurse	Sch.N ass.	Fam. Plan.	Comm. Psych.	Geria-tric	Liai-son	Clinic
	%	%	%	%	%	%	%	%	%	%	%	%	%	%	%	%	%	%
(i) Technical tests, assessments, screening and surveillance:																		
Clinics	†	†	†	†	†	†	67	25	25	50	65	78	36	85	†	†	†	87
Home visits							3	71	72	40	3	1	1	1				2
Other							30	4	3	10	32	21	63	14				11
Average hours spent on technical tests (= 100%)	*0.4*	*0.5*	*0.5*	*0.2*	*0.4*	*0.4*	*2.3*	*6.7*	*2.1*	*1.7*	*3.2*	*7.1*	*9.9*	*1.9*	*0.1*	*0.3*	*0.2*	*4.2*
(ii) Technical procedures:																		
Clinics	10	12	10	5	3	†	64	4	6	†	86	63	22	†	9	–	43	76
Home visits	84	82	82	89	90		1	45	89		*	*	–		57	87	34	2
Other	6	6	8	6	7		35	51	5		14	37	78		34	13	23	22
Average hours spent on technical procedures (= 100%)	*6.5*	*6.6*	*5.1*	*8.0*	*7.0*	*0.5*	*3.6*	*1.2*	*5.3*	*0.2*	*1.2*	*1.6*	*0.9*	*0.2*	*1.0*	*1.0*	*1.4*	*4.0*
(iii) Other nursing care:																		
Clinics	*	*	*	*	–	1	†	1	*	†	32	59	30	73	13	–	*	56
Home visits	97	97	98	98	94	97		79	97		39	9	*	12	54	89	85	39
Other	3	3	2	2	6	2		20	3		29	32	70	15	33	11	15	5
Average hours spent on other nursing care (= 100%)	*6.3*	*6.2*	*4.8*	*7.8*	*7.9*	*13.1*	*0.4*	*2.1*	*4.8*	*0.4*	*1.0*	*1.4*	*2.4*	*0.7*	*1.5*	*4.0*	*1.4*	*1.4*
(iv) Advice, counselling, reassurance and education:																		
Clinics	1	2	3	1	*	3	52	20	9	22	18	40	12	78	6	4	14	36
Home visits	92	92	88	94	96	91	9	73	88	68	69	29	36	4	73	89	42	48
Other	7	6	9	5	4	6	39	7	3	10	13	31	52	18	21	7	44	16
Average hours spent on advisory activities (= 100%)	*2.8*	*2.9*	*2.3*	*2.8*	*2.3*	*1.1*	*1.2*	*5.5*	*3.2*	*9.1*	*4.1*	*2.5*	*1.0*	*2.6*	*10.3*	*6.4*	*6.2*	*2.0*
Number of nurses	736	410	158	116	52	541	252	313	91	967	63	409	35	202	117	39	48	48

† Proportions have not been calculated where nurses spent half an hour or less on a particular area of activity.

and greater proportions on technical tests and procedures. They also spent some time on school clinics—both hearing and vision, and school medicals—where technical tests and assessments took up most of the time.

School nurses and *school nurse assistants* spent the greater part of their clinic time on school clinics doing technical tests and assessments. *GP employed nurses* spent the greatest proportion of time amongst the different types of nurses on technical procedures—49%. *Clinic nurses* had a similar pattern to GP employed nurses for the GP surgery sessions they did but they also did clinics connected with young children and in these had a pattern more like health visitor assistants. Their overall proportions are therefore a combination of the two patterns.

9.6 Time with patients excluding clinics

Table 9.8 shows the proportions of time spent with patients, excluding clinics on the four main areas of activity. All the types of nurses have been included but some, such as family planning and GP employed nurses,

spent only a small amount of time with patients outside clinics. We have seen that for district nurses and auxiliaries time with patients that is not spent in clinics is largely spent on home visits but for some types of nurses other patient contacts—visits to schools, hospitals etc—are more common.

Many of the variations between the different types of nurses were also apparent in Table 9.2 (which was based on all time with patients, including clinics) and were commented on then. The two tables are obviously very similar for those types of nurses who did not spend much time on clinics. For the other types of nurses it is interesting to compare Tables 9.7 and 9.8. Midwives, for instance, had a different pattern of work in clinics compared to home visits and other patient contacts. In clinics they spent just over half of their time on technical tests and assessments (Table 9.7) whereas only 37% of their other time with patients was spent on these activities (Table 9.8). Greater proportions of their other time with patients were spent on technical procedures and other nursing care.

Table 9.7 Proportion of time in clinics spent on different areas of activity, by type of nurse

Area of activity	Mid-wives	DN/Midw.	HV	HV ass.	Schl. Nurse	Sch.N ass.	GP empl.	Fam. Plan.	Liai-son	Clinic
	%	%	%	%	%	%	%	%	%	%
Technical tests, assessments and surveillance	52	34	27	45	65	75	33	39	6	46
Technical procedures	1	20	3	22	12	4	49	4	37	35
Other nursing care	1	2	1	7	9	15	4	11	*	9
Advice, counselling, reassurance and education	34	17	60	17	11	2	13	46	49	9
Unspecified	12	27	9	9	3	4	1	*	8	1
Average hours spent on clinics (= 100%)	*3.3*	*1.6*	*3.2*	*4.5*	*8.9*	*5.8*	*4.6*	*3.9*	*1.7*	*7.4*
Number of nurses	313	91	967	63	409	35	252	202	48	48

Table 9.8 Proportion of time with patients (excluding clinics) spent on the different areas of activity, by type of nurse

Area of activity	All DNs	DN SRN+	DN SRN−	DN SEN+	DN SEN−	Auxil-iaries	GP empl.	Mid-wives	DN/Midw.	HV	HV ass.	Schl. Nurse	Sch.N ass.	Fam. Plan.	Comm. Psych.	Geria-tric	Liai-son	Clinic
	%	%	%	%	%	%	%	%	%	%	%	%	%	%	%	%	%	%
Technical tests, assessments and surveillance	2	2	2	1	2	1	26	37	11	10	18	32	62	23	1	1	1	17
Technical procedures	58	37	37	41	39	3	44	9	33	2	4	13	7	5	7	8	10	29
Other nursing care	40	39	40	41	45	87	5	15	32	3	11	12	17	14	10	33	18	15
Advice, counselling, reassurance and education	17	18	18	15	13	7	20	32	20	77	54	30	8	47	78	50	66	27
Unspecified	3	4	3	2	1	2	5	7	4	8	13	13	6	11	4	8	5	12
Average hours spent with patients excluding clinics (= 100%)	*15.7*	*15.6*	*12.4*	*18.8*	*17.1*	*14.8*	*3.1*	*13.6*	*15.0*	*9.3*	*6.1*	*4.6*	*9.2*	*1.7*	*12.3*	*12.2*	*8.1*	*4.8*
Number of nurses	736	410	158	116	52	541	252	313	91	967	63	409	35	202	117	39	48	48

10 Non-nursing activity

In Chapter 6 we saw that most types of nurses working in the community spent a quarter or more of their working time on non-clinical or non-nursing activities. This chapter looks in more detail at the various non-clinical activities that nurses carried out, when they were not with patients. The nine categories of non-clinical activity used in the diary are listed below.

NON-CLINICAL ACTIVITIES
01 No access visit, waiting, no reply
02 Clerical and administrative related to own job:
    Filing, checking clerical data
    Mileage claims
    Kalamazoo
    Work list, work plan
    Write letters
    Survey time
03 Clerical and administrative related to clients/patients:
    Requests for equipment, aids, prescriptions, services etc
    Clients'/patients' reports
    Clients'/patients' notes
    Client/patient register
04 Telephone calls
05 Meeting/consultation/liaison visits/case conference/ court appearance
06 Training, teaching, supervision (given/received):
    Own training—in service
    Study time, course, conference, research, discussions with supervisor
    Teaching/supervision—aides, auxiliaries, students and student reports
07 Preparation and collection of equipment, supplies, uniform, car etc
08 Reception duty (GP nurses)
09 Other non-clinical (specify)

10.1 Proportion of time spent on each non-clinical activity

The proportion of average working time spent on non-clinical activities by the different types of nurses varied considerably, from 16% for auxiliaries to 57% for GP employed practice nurses (see Table 6.4). When time spent on travel was excluded, the proportion of activity time spent on non-clinical activities varied even more (see Table 9.1). Table 10.1 shows the proportion of activity time spent on all non-clinical activities and the proportion of activity time spent on each of the nine non-clinical activities. Auxiliaries spent the lowest proportion, 20%, of their activity time on non-clinical activities and GP employed practice nurses and liaison nurses the highest, with 58% and 67% respectively. District nurses and midwives spent approximately one third of their time doing non-clinical activities and for health visitors and most other types of nurses the proportion was around one half. Amongst district nursing staff those who were less qualified spent a lower proportion of their time on non-clinical activities—the proportion ranged from 37% for district nurse SRNs with a district nursing qualification to 28% for district nurse SENs without a district nursing qualification and 20% for auxiliaries. Although auxiliaries had such a low proportion, health visitor and school nurse assistants did not follow the same pattern. They spent 53% and 47% respectively on non-clinical activities.

Clerical and administrative work related to the nurse's job and to patients were the activities on which most types of nurses spent a lot of their time—from 12% for auxiliaries to 35% for school nurse assistants. There were some variations in the proportion of time the different types of nurses spent on particular non-clinical activities. These variations are more easily seen in Table 10.2, which shows the time spent on each of the non-clinical activities as a

Table 10.1 Proportion of activity time spent on the various non-clinical activities, by type of nurse

Activities	All DNs	DN SRN+	DN SRN−	DN SEN+	DN SEN−	Auxil-iaries	GP empl.	Mid-wives	DN/ Midw.	HV	HV ass.	Schl. Nurse	Sch.N ass.	Fam. Plan.	Comm. Psych.	Geria-tric	Liai-son	Clinic
	%	%	%	%	%	%	%	%	%	%	%	%	%	%	%	%	%	%
No access, waiting	1	1	1	1	1	1	2	1	1	2	1	1	*	1	1	1	1	2
Clerical and administrative related to nurse's job	12 }19	13 }20	12 }19	12 }19	11 }17	7 }12	9 }26	13 }20	13 }18	16 }30	14 }31	14 }27	19 }35	5 }15	10 }21	15 }29	10 }23	13 }30
Clerical and administrative related to patients	7	7	7	7	6	5	17	7	5	14	17	13	16	10	11	14	13	17
Telephone calls	5	6	4	5	3	2	6	7	6	7	5	4	2	3	5	8	12	4
Meetings	5	5	4	4	2	1	3	3	5	8	5	6	2	2	14	6	23	3
Training, teaching etc.	2	2	5	1	3	1	*	3	6	5	3	4	2	6	8	3	4	1
Preparation of equipment etc.	2	2	2	2	2	2	3	2	2	2	5	4	3	12	1	1	1	6
Reception duty	*	*	*	*	*	*	16	*	*	*	1	*	−	2	*	−	*	1
Other non-clinical	1	1	*	*	*	1	2	1	1	1	2	2	3	1	2	1	3	1
All non-clinical activities	35	37	35	32	28	20	58	37	39	55	53	48	47	42	52	49	67	48
Activities with patients (including unspecified)	65	63	65	68	72	80	42	63	61	45	47	52	53	58	48	51	33	52
Average activity hours *(= 100%)*	25.5	26.8	20.2	28.4	24.0	19.4	18.4	26.9	27.2	27.5	22.4	25.9	28.4	9.8	28.1	24.5	29.8	23.2
Number of nurses	736	410	158	116	52	541	252	313	91	967	63	409	35	202	117	39	48	48

proportion of the time spent on all non-clinical activities only. Training is discussed separately, in Section 10.2.

Looking first at *district nurses*, all four types of district nurse spent around 20% of their non-clinical time on clerical and administrative activities related to patients and around a third on clerical and administrative activities related to their own job. District nurse SENs, however, spent a higher proportion of their time than SRNs on the latter activity, 39% compared to 34%. SENs who did not have a district nursing qualification spent only six per cent of their time on meetings compared to 12% to 14% for other district nurses. Both SRNs and SENs without a district nursing qualification spent a greater proportion of time—twice as much—on training than those with a qualification. The code for training included both that given and that received so we cannot separate the time spent on these two aspects of training. However the majority of time spent on training was probably spent on training received (see Section 10.2) and it is not therefore surprising that those without a district nursing qualification spent a greater proportion of their time receiving training.

Auxiliaries had a similar pattern to district nurses but spent a slightly greater proportion of their time on preparation and collection of equipment etc and less on telephone calls and meetings. They spent only a small proportion of time—three per cent—on training. *GP employed practice nurses* spent 28% of their non-clinical time on reception duty and, unlike most nurses, spent a greater proportion of time on clerical and administrative work related to patients (30%) than on clerical and administrative work related to their job (15%).

Midwives and district nurse/midwives also had a similar pattern to district nurses although midwives spent a larger proportion of time on telephone calls. *Health visitors and assistants and school nurses and assistants* all spent a larger proportion of time than district nurses and midwives on clerical and administrative activities related to patients, particularly the assistants who both spent 33% of their time on this. *School nurse assistants* spent 40% on clerical and administrative activities related to their own job. The assistants spent less time on meetings than health visitors and school nurses.

Family planning nurses spent the largest proportion of time—29%—on preparation and collection of equipment and a smaller proportion of time than other types of nurses—12%—on clerical activities related to their job. *Community psychiatric and liaison nurses* spent the largest proportions of time amongst the different types of nurses on meetings—28% and 33% respectively.

Turning now to work organisation, there was little variation between nurses with different work organisation patterns. We saw in Chapter 6 (Table 6.6) that there were no differences between attached and not attached nurses in the proportion of time spent on non-clinical activities except for auxiliaries where the attached did a smaller proportion than the not attached. Table 10.3 shows, for the four main types of nurses, the proportions of time spent by attached and not attached nurses on the various non-clinical activities. There were no significant differences for district nurses and midwives. Attached health visitors and auxiliaries spent a higher proportion of time than the not attached on clerical and administrative work related to their own job. As attached district nurses and midwives spent slightly higher proportions of time than their not attached counterparts on clerical and administrative work related to their own job we compared the proportions of time spent on this activity by all attached and not attached nurses, that is, the four types of nurses added together. The attached did have a slightly higher proportion—33% compared to 30%—but the difference was not significant.

There were some other differences between attached and not attached auxiliaries—in particular, auxiliaries who were not attached spent a greater proportion of time on preparation of equipment and 'other' non-clinical activities. However auxiliaries did spend less time and a smaller proportion of their time on non-clinical activities than the other three types of nurses so these differences are based on only small variations in the absolute time.

There was no pattern of variation between nurses working with different numbers of practices for any of the four types of nurses.

10.2 Training
The code which was used in the diary for 'training' included both training given, that is teaching and

Table 10.2 Proportion of non-clinical time spent on the various non-clinical activities, by type of nurse

Activities	All DNs	DN SRN+	DN SRN-	DN SEN+	DN SEN-	Auxil-iaries	GP empl.	Mid-wives	DN/ Midw.	HV	HV ass.	Schl. Nurse	Sch.N ass.	Fam. Plan.	Comm. Psych.	Geria-tric	Liai-son	Clinic
	%	%	%	%	%	%	%	%	%	%	%	%	%	%	%	%	%	%
No access, waiting	3	3	3	2	2	3	3	3	2	3	2	2	1	3	1	3	1	5
Clerical and administrative related to nurse's job	35	35	33	39	39	35	15	35	34	29	27	29	40	12	20	31	15	28
Clerical and administrative related to patients	20	19	20	21	21	24	30	19	14	26	33	28	33	23	21	28	20	35
Telephone calls	14	15	12	14	12	8	11	18	15	13	8	8	5	6	10	16	18	9
Meetings	13	14	12	13	6	8	4	10	12	14	9	12	4	5	28	12	33	5
Training, teaching etc.	7	6	13	3	12	3	1	7	14	8	6	7	4	14	15	6	6	1
Preparation of equipment etc	6	6	5	7	6	11	4	6	6	4	10	9	7	29	2	2	2	12
Reception duty	*	*	*	*	*	*	28	*	*	*	1	1	–	5	*	–	*	3
Other	2	2	2	1	2	8	4	2	3	3	4	4	6	3	3	2	5	2
Average hours spent on non-clinical activities (=100%)	*8.9*	*9.8*	*7.0*	*9.1*	*6.9*	*4.0*	*10.7*	*10.0*	*10.5*	*15.0*	*11.7*	*12.4*	*13.5*	*4.2*	*14.6*	*11.9*	*20.0*	*11.1*
Number of nurses	736	410	158	116	52	541	252	313	91	967	63	409	35	202	117	39	48	48

supervision, and training received. As mentioned already this means that we cannot separate the time spent on these two different aspects of training. When the pilot study for the survey was carried out, however, there were two separate codes—one for training given and one for training received. Analysis of the pilot study showed that so little time was spent on 'training given' that it was not worth having a separate code. It is therefore reasonable to assume that almost all of the time recorded under the training code was spent on training received.

A small percentage of nurses attended a training course or conference during their week of diary recording. Table 10.4 shows the proportion of nurses who spent one day or more away from work attending a training course or conference. Overall four per cent of nurses working in the community spent at least one day at a course or conference. The highest proportions were 12% for joint duty district nurse/midwives and nine per cent for community psychiatric nurses and district nurse SRNs without a district nursing qualification. Table 10.2 showed that district nurses without a district nursing qualification spent twice as much time on training as those with a qualification and Table 10.4 supports this conclusion in relation to attendance of training courses.

It seemed likely that the time that these nurses spent on the courses accounted for a large part of the time spent on training overall. This was confirmed when the proportion of activity time spent on training by nurses who attended courses was compared with the proportion spent by those who had not attended courses. Training accounted for a much larger proportion of the time of nurses who had been on a course—22% for district nurses, for example, compared with two per cent for nurses who had not attended courses. Of the nurses who had not attended a course, community psychiatric nurses spent five per cent of their activity time on training and health visitors four per cent. All the other kinds of nurses spent three per cent or less of their time on training.

10.3 Non-clinical activity in the nurses' homes

Table 10.5 shows the proportion of non-clinical activities which were carried out in the nurses' own homes. All types of district nurses, midwives and joint duty district nurse/midwives did at least two fifths of their non-clinical work at home and auxiliaries did 29%. We saw in Chapter 3 (Table 3.8) that a large proportion of these types of nurses worked from home* and they often used their

*Q17 Where do you work from on a daily basis?

Table 10.3 Proportion of non-clinical time spent on the various non-clinical activities, by attachment

Type of non-clinical activity	District nurses		Midwives		Health visitors		Auxiliaries	
	Not attached	Attached	Not attached	Attached	Not attached	Attached	Not attached	Attached
	%	%	%	%	%	%	%	%
No access, waiting	5	2	4	3	2	3	2	3
Clerical and administrative related to nurse's job	33	36	33	36	24	30	31	40
Clerical and administrative related to patients	22	20	18	19	28	26	27	23
Telephone calls	15	14	18	18	14	13	6	11
Meetings	11	14	10	9	14	14	4	11
Training, teaching etc	5	7	8	7	9	8	1	4
Preparation of equipment etc	6	6	6	6	4	4	18	6
Other (including reception duty)	3	1	3	2	5	2	11	2
Average hours spent on non-clinical activities (= 100%)	*7.8*	*9.5*	*10.7*	*10.3*	*15.2*	*15.2*	*5.1*	*3.3*
Number of nurses	111	529	53	237	106	835	140	314

Table 10.4 Attendance of training courses, by type of nurse

	All DNs	DN SRN+	DN SRN-	DN SEN+	DN SEN-	Auxil-iaries	GP empl.	Mid-wives	DN/ Midw.	HV	HV ass.	Schl. Nurse	Sch.N ass.	Fam. Plan.	Comm. Psych.	Geria-tric	Liai-son	Clinic
Proportion of nurses who had one day or more attending a course	5%	4%	9%	2%	4%	1%	1%	4%	12%	4%	2%	4%	–	3%	9%	–	2%	–
*Number of nurses (= 100%)†	699*	*390*	*152*	*108*	*49*	*487*	*229*	*300*	*81*	*893*	*59*	*381*	*33*	*179*	*110*	*37*	*44*	*46*

† Bases are smaller than usual because some nurses had not always recorded whether or not they were at work and they were excluded from the analysis.

Table 10.5 Proportion of time spent on non-clinical activities in nurse's home, by type of nurse

Location	All DNs	DN SRN+	DN SRN-	DN SEN+	DN SEN-	Auxil-iaries	GP empl.	Mid-wives	DN/ Midw.	HV	HV ass.	Schl. Nurse	Sch.N ass.	Fam. Plan.	Comm. Psych.	Geria-tric	Liai-son	Clinic
	%	%	%	%	%	%	%	%	%	%	%	%	%	%	%	%	%	%
Nurse's own home	40	39	41	45	38	29	2	55	56	9	3	8	3	5	7	10	9	3
Other location	60	61	59	55	62	71	98	45	44	91	97	92	97	95	93	90	91	97
Average hours spent on non-clinical activities (= 100%)	*8.9*	*9.8*	*7.0*	*9.1*	*6.9*	*4.0*	*10.7*	*10.0*	*10.5*	*15.0*	*11.7*	*12.4*	*13.5*	*4.2*	*14.6*	*11.9*	*20.0*	*11.1*
Number of nurses	736	410	158	116	52	541	252	313	91	967	63	409	35	202	117	39	48	48

home as an office or at least received and made telephone calls from home. The other types of nurses did only small proportions—between two and ten per cent—of their non-clinical work at home. The rest of the section concentrates, therefore, on the four types of nurses who did a substantial part of their non-clinical work at home.

Table 10.6 compares the proportion of non-clinical activities carried out at home by nurses who worked from home with that of those who did not. The table confirms that nurses who worked from home carried out a larger proportion of their non-clinical work at home than nurses who were based elsewhere. However even the latter group did a considerable minority of their non-clinical work at home.

Most of the non-clinical work that nurses did in their own homes was either clerical and administrative work (both related to their own job and related to patients) or telephone calls. Table 10.7 shows the proportion of each of these three activities which was carried out in nurses' homes, for nurses who worked from home and for those who did not. Nurses of all four types who worked from home did 70% or more of the clerical and administrative work related to their job at home, with midwives and district nurse/midwives doing the highest proportions. Apart from auxiliaries, even those who were not based at home did around half of this work at home. Rather

lower proportions of clerical and administrative work related to patients were carried out at home—only joint duty district nurse/midwives did more than half of this work at home. All types of nurses apart from auxiliaries not working from home did large proportions of their telephoning from home—the proportions ranged from 48% for district nurses not working from home to 86% for home-based midwives.

10.4 Assistance with clerical work

Chapter 3 included a section on assistance with clerical work which showed that there was a wide variation between different types of nurses in the proportion who could call on help with their clerical work. The groups of staff where large proportions worked from home—district nurses, midwives and joint duty staff—were less likely to have clerical assistance. Table 10.8 shows the proportions of time spent on clerical and administrative work and on all non-clinical activities by the different types of nurses, according to whether or not they had clerical assistance. When all types of nurses are considered together (in the last two columns of the table) it is clear that nurses *with* clerical assistance spent a greater proportion of their time than nurses with no help on both non-clinical activities and on clerical and administrative work related to patients.

Table 10.6 Proportion of time spent on non-clinical activities in nurses' homes, by whether nurse worked from home

Location for non-clinical activities	District nurses		Midwives		DN/Midwives		Auxiliaries	
	Works from home	Other	Works from home	Other	Works from home	Other	Works from home	Other
	%	%	%	%	%	%	%	%
Nurse's own home	47	29	58	27	57	47	47	11
Other location	53	71	42	73	43	53	53	89
Average hours spent on non-clinical activities (= 100%)	*9.0*	*8.8*	*10.1*	*9.4*	*10.4*	*11.2*	*3.0*	*6.1*
Number of nurses	465	267	277	36	78	12	366	173

Table 10.7 Proportion of time spent on the non-clinical activities most commonly carried out at home

Type of non-clinical activity	District nurses		Midwives		DN/Midwives		Auxiliaries	
	Works from home	Other	Works from home	Other	Works from home	Other	Works from home	Other
Clerical and administrative related to nurse's job								
Proportion of time spent on them at home	73%	49%	85%	49%	87%	69%	72%	25%
Average hours spent on them at all locations (= 100%)	*3.2*	*3.1*	*3.6*	*2.8*	*3.6*	*3.6*	*1.2*	*1.8*
Clerical and administrative related to patients								
Proportion of time spent on them at home	30%	15%	37%	12%	50%	54%	26%	7%
Average hours spent on them at all locations (= 100%)	*1.7*	*1.9*	*1.8*	*2.4*	*1.5*	*1.3*	*0.6*	*1.6*
Telephone calls								
Proportion of time spent on them at home	71%	48%	86%	55%	78%	61%	84%	27%
Average hours spent on them at all locations (= 100%)	*1.4*	*1.0*	*2.0*	*0.9*	*1.6*	*1.4*	*0.4*	*0.2*
Number of nurses	465	267	277	36	78	12	366	173

Table 10.8 Proportion of time spent on clerical work and non-clinical activities, by nurses with and without clerical assistance †

Type of activity	All DNs		GP empl.		Midwives		HV		Schl. Nurse		Fam. Plan.		Comm. Psych.		Geriatric		Liaison		Clinic		All Nurses	
	Cl. ass	No. ass	Cl. ass	No ass	Cl. ass	No ass	Cl ass	No ass	Cl. ass	No ass	Cl. ass	No ass	Cl. ass	No ass	Cl. ass	No ass	Cl. ass	No ass	Cl. ass	No ass	Cl. ass	No ass
	%	%	%	%	%	%	%	%	%	%	%	%	%	%	%	%	%	%	%	%	%	%
Clerical and administrative related to own job	13	13	8	12	13	13	15	17	14	14	5	5	10	11	17	15	10	10	9	12	13	13
Clerical and administrative related to patients	8	7	18	17	10	7	15	14	14	12	10	9	11	11	11	16	19	11	19	14	13	9
All non-clinical activities	37	36	58	60	42	37	55	55	50	45	40	48	52	52	46	53	69	68	45	45	51	42
Average activity hours (= 100%)	26.9	25.9	18.6	18.2	34.9	27.4	27.0	28.7	26.5	25.5	9.7	10.5	27.4	29.2	19.1	26.0	26.7	31.4	23.4	23.2	24.2	26.0
Number of nurses ††	189	1089	170	80	17	274	540	403	202	200	134	62	69	48	12	32	15	32	23	21	1373	2324

† Auxiliaries, health visitor assistants and school nurse assistants were not asked whether they had clerical assistance. Only two district nurse/midwives had clerical assistance so joint duty staff have also been excluded from the table.

†† Bases are smaller because full-time relief nurses were not asked about clerical assistance.

11 The 24 health districts—similarities and differences

This chapter draws together findings from Chapters 2, 3, 5 and 7 and gives data on some of the main survey variables for each of the 24 health districts which were included in the survey. It aims to describe the variation between the districts and to explore relationships between the survey variables and some characteristics of the districts.

11.1 Types of nurses employed in health districts

Table 11.1 shows for each of the 24 health districts the number of nurses working in the community in post at the time of the survey and their distribution between the different types of nurses. It includes the five per cent of nurses who were not contacted during the survey period or who refused to take part. These nurses were assigned to the broad groups provided by health authorities for sampling purposes. Since only one half of the district nurses working in the districts were included their numbers have been doubled in this table to give a true representation of the distribution of different kinds of staff.

In the right hand column of Table 11.1 it can be seen that 33% of all nurses working in the community were district nurses and 21% were health visitors (20%) or their assistants (1%). Midwives and district nurse/midwives accounted for another ten per cent of staff; auxiliaries for 11%. The school nursing service accounted for nine per cent of staff and family planning for four per cent. Six per cent of the nurses were employed directly by general practitioners and three per cent were community psychiatric nurses. Geriatric, liaison and clinic nurses between them accounted for the last three per cent of staff.

Joint duty district nurse/midwives have been generally phased out but were found in six of the 24 health districts. In the districts in which they were found joint duty staff tended to be as numerous as single duty midwives. This may imply a definite policy of keeping joint duty staff.

Midwives were found in all districts although there was a wide variation in the proportion of all staff that they comprised—from three per cent to 16%. Much of this variation was probably due to the different arrangements that districts make for dividing midwifery between hospital and community.

District nurses were the largest group in all the districts but again, like midwives, the proportion they comprised was extremely variable. In one district only 25% of the staff were district nurses—in two others 42% were in this category.

There was also a large variation in the proportion of staff who were *auxiliaries*. One district had none, in the others the proportion who were auxiliaries varied from six per cent to 17%.

Table 11.1 Types of nurses employed by health districts—based on number of staff in post

Type of nurse	District† 1	2	3	4	5	6	7	8	9	10	11	12	13	14	15	16	17	18	19	20	21	22	23	24	All
	%	%	%	%	%	%	%	%	%	%	%	%	%	%	%	%	%	%	%	%	%	%	%	%	%
DN SRN+	23	11	14	14	24	16	16	14	14	20	16	14	24	11	16	17	24	13	20	13	19	16	16	20	17
DN SRN–	6	7	6	4	8	6	6	12	5	6	7	4	7	7	9	4	1	5	4	7	3	18	3	5	6
DN SEN+	2	4	6	3	4	9	3	1	7	6	5	2	9	4	–	4	4	8	7	3	4	6	12	6	5
DN SEN–	9	4	3	–	2	3	2	–	1	6	3	3	–	5	6	4	2	2	2	5	–	1	2	2	3
DN NR††	1	4	–	6	2	2	5	1	1	3	–	2	1	2	–	4	2	1	9	–	*	1	2	2	2
All district nurses	41	30	29	27	40	36	32	28	28	41	31	25	41	29	31	33	33	29	42	28	26	42	35	35	33
Midwives	9	3	3	4	6	4	13	5	10	5	1	9	9	10	2	5	10	5	16	7	6	10	10	7	8
District nurse/ midwives	–	11	–	–	–	–	–	7	–	–	9	–	3	–	14	–	–	–	–	7	–	–	–	–	2
Health visitors	19	19	19	18	19	18	23	19	22	19	22	21	25	24	18	17	22	26	19	25	16	21	20	21	20
HV assistant	*	1	3	–	1	*	–	*	1	1	–	6	2	*	–	1	1	*	–	6	1	*	–	2	1
Auxiliaries etc	13	7	14	7	13	17	7	10	12	6	12	14	–	12	13	17	10	9	7	12	16	10	16	13	11
GP employed nurses	1	9	1	8	6	8	5	14	9	2	6	12	9	4	9	11	10	1	1	4	5	3	1	6	6
School nurses	11	11	10	14	4	5	15	3	7	12	8	2	3	12	8	7	6	19	10	4	14	7	6	5	8
School N assistant	–	1	–	1	–	1	–	–	3	–	–	–	–	–	–	–	–	–	–	3	2	3	1	1	1
Family planning	–	4	9	3	5	5	3	6	6	9	2	7	7	5	–	4	4	6	2	4	6	2	2	6	4
Community psychiatric	2	2	3	3	3	1	*	5	1	3	9	3	–	–	4	2	3	1	2	2	3	2	5	2	3
Geriatric nurses	1	1	–	14	–	–	–	1	1	*	–	–	–	*	1	2	–	*	–	–	3	–	2	–	1
Liaison nurses	1	–	2	1	2	1	*	1	*	2	–	1	2	*	1	–	1	1	–	1	1	*	2	1	1
Clinic nurses	2	1	7	1	–	5	2	1	–	1	–	*	1	2	*	–	1	3	–	1	–	–	*	–	1
Number of nurses (= 100%)	211	226	201	132	272	225	227	178	336	207	208	234	176	270	270	116	184	126	217	137	346	297	223	382	5401

†The district numbers on this and following tables are those used to identify them for data processing.

††NR denotes non-responding district nurses. Since the tables are based on staff in post it is necessary to include those who refused to be interviewed or who were not contacted. We knew which type of nurse these were except for the non-responding district nurses who are shown as a separate category because their qualifications were not known.

Health visitors, the second largest group of staff, were however found in all districts in much more consistent proportions. They comprised between 16% and 26% of staff. Eighteen districts employed health visitor assistants. They comprised between one and six per cent of the total number of staff.

All districts had a *school nursing service* although in some districts school nurses made up a very small proportion of staff. This may have been because the service was mainly provided by health visitors.

All but two districts had some *family planning nurses;* all but two had some *community psychiatric nurses*.

The other types of nurses—*geriatric, liaison and clinic*—were found in fewer of the districts. For example only half had specialist geriatric nurses and two districts accounted for 62% of all the geriatric nurses identified. Similarly only 15 districts had clinic nurses, two districts accounting for 48% of all those found.

Table 11.2 is similar to Table 11.1 except that it is based on the estimated full-time equivalents of staff in post rather than their actual numbers. These estimates were calculated by counting staff who worked less than 11 hours per week as one quarter, those who worked 11–30 hours as one half and those who worked 31 or more hours

as full-time. As can be seen from the total column the proportion of staff who were district nurses rises to 35% and that of health visitors to 25%. These two major groups of staff are of course usually employed full-time. Other groups who are often part-time staff show as a smaller proportion of total staff. This applies to auxiliaries, GP employed practice nurses and family planning nurses.

Table 11.3 shows the proportions of district nurses and health visitors in each district who were employed on a part-time basis. As can be seen there was much variation between districts for both types of staff. Two districts (3 and 4) employed no part-time district nurses whilst 37% of District 16 district nurses were part-time and 50% of those in District 22. The variation was not quite so extreme for health visitors. There were no part-timers in District 6 but 35% of those in District 10 worked part-time.

Fewer than one half of the districts had broadly similar rates of part-time working for both types of staff. For example District 6 had very low rates and District 22 very high rates. Among the majority of districts there was little relationship implying that if recruitment of part-time district nurses and health visitors was part of a definite policy the policy was rather different for the two types of staff.

Table 11.2 Types of nurses employed by health district—based on full-time equivalents of staff in post†

Type of nurse	District																								
	1	2	3	4	5	6	7	8	9	10	11	12	13	14	15	16	17	18	19	20	21	22	23	24	All
	%	%	%	%	%	%	%	%	%	%	%	%	%	%	%	%	%	%	%	%	%	%	%	%	%
District nurses	42	31	32	29	43	41	35	32	32	44	35	29	43	31	31	33	35	36	42	32	29	39	39	38	35
Midwives	10	4	3	3	8	5	14	7	12	6	1	11	10	11	3	7	11	7	17	8	7	11	10	9	8
District nurse/ midwives	–	14	–	–	–	–	–	8	–	–	11	–	3	–	17	–	–	–	–	7	–	–	–	–	2
Health visitors††	22	22	22	19	22	22	24	23	25	22	26	31	30	27	22	29	26	30	19	33	18	24	20	27	25
Auxiliaries	9	5	14	7	10	17	6	6	9	6	7	10	–	13	9	10	7	6	8	11	17	7	10	8	9
GP employed nurses	*	6	1	8	4	5	4	9	6	2	3	9	5	2	7	7	8	1	1	2	4	4	1	4	4
School nurses††	10	13	11	14	5	3	14	3	11	10	5	3	4	10	6	5	7	13	10	3	15	10	11	6	9
Family planning	–	2	4	1	2	2	1	2	3	5	1	2	4	2	–	1	2	2	*	2	2	1	2	3	2
Community psychiatric	2	3	3	3	4	1	*	6	2	3	11	4	–	–	5	3	4	2	2	2	4	3	5	3	3
Geriatric nurses	1	*	–	14	–	–	–	3	–	*	–	–	–	*	*	3	–	–	–	–	3	–	2	–	1
Liaison nurses	2	–	2	1	2	1	*	1	*	2	–	–	1	2	*	1	–	1	1	–	1	1	*	2	1
Clinic nurses	2	*	8	1	–	3	2	*	–	–	–	*	1	–	2	*	1	*	2	–	*	–	–	*	1
Number of full-time equivalents (= 100%)	*169*	*187*	*175*	*121*	*219*	*193*	*195*	*141*	*268*	*165*	*171*	*172*	*151*	*218*	*223*	*86*	*160*	*95*	*198*	*112*	*304*	*215*	*195*	*310*	*4443*

†Full-time equivalents were calculated by counting staff who worked less than 11 hours per week as one quarter, those who worked 11–30 hours as one half and those who worked 31 or more hours as full-time. The small number of non-responders were weighted with the average for their particular type of nurse in their district.
††Including assistants.

Table 11.3 Full and part-time† working amongst district nurses and health visitors

	District																								
	1	2	3	4	5	6	7	8	9	10	11	12	13	14	15	16	17	18	19	20	21	22	23	24	All
Proportion of district nurses working part-time	28%	20%	—	—	17%	1%	10%	15%	13%	29%	12%	27%	17%	19%	29%	37%	7%	12%	15%	11%	3%	50%	6%	20%	18%
Number of district nurses (= 100%)	*41*	*30*	*28*	*14*	*52*	*38*	*30*	*24*	*45*	*40*	*32*	*26*	*34*	*36*	*40*	*16*	*28*	*17*	*34*	*18*	*44*	*59*	*36*	*62*	*824*
Proportion of health visitors working part-time	13%	7%	17%	13%	21%	—	21%	9%	25%	35%	11%	18%	10%	23%	8%	16%	10%	30%	11%	12%	20%	34%	21%	15%	17%
Numbers of health visitors (= 100%)	*38*	*41*	*36*	*23*	*47*	*39*	*52*	*33*	*72*	*34*	*47*	*44*	*37*	*48*	*44*	*16*	*35*	*23*	*33*	*29*	*44*	*38*	*34*	*69*	*1056*

†Part-time working is 30 hours or less per week.

66

The district nursing service

Table 11.4 is similar to Table 11.2 but looks at district nurses and auxiliaries in much more detail. The main purpose of the table is to look at the variation in employment of staff with different qualifications. Joint duty staff are not therefore included although the six districts which employed them are indicated.

As can be seen from the total column of Table 11.2 district nurses and auxiliaries comprise 44% of the full-time equivalent staff of all districts. Of these staff Table 11.4 shows that 43% were district nurse SRNs with district training. For 17 of the districts this proportion fell between 37% and 47%. There were two districts (6 and 14) which had a particularly low proportion of such highly trained staff—32% and 31% respectively. In contrast 60% of District 17's staff were in this category and 62% of staff in District 13. None of the districts employed no SENs but four of them employed no SENs without district training. The district (13) with the highest proportion of the most highly trained district nurses employed no auxiliaries at all—apart from that district they comprised between 12% and 37% of staff in the district nursing service.

District nurses and auxiliaries spend the majority of their time caring for the elderly. It might therefore be expected that the proportion of such staff in a district was related to the proportion of the elderly among the population of the district. However there appeared to be no such relationship. But as we have seen from Tables 11.1 and 11.2 some districts have other groups of staff who spend much of their time with the elderly—in particular joint duty district nurse/midwives and geriatric nurses. From Tables 8.2 and 8.5 it seems reasonable to assume that joint duty staff spend approximately three quarters of their time on district nurse work. A more complete estimate of numbers of staff who work mainly with the elderly, is therefore obtained by adding three quarters of the joint duty staff and all the geriatric nurses to the full-time equivalent numbers of district nurses and auxiliaries. When this is done these groups of staff account for 47% of the full-time equivalents of nurses working in the community. The proportion ranges from 38% in District 20 to 58% in District 6.

The relationship between the proportion of staff who mainly care for the elderly and the proportion of elderly among the districts' population is explored in Table 11.5.

Column d indicates those districts where the proportion of elderly in the population is greater than the average for the 24 districts†. As can be seen, in general, the districts where the proportion of staff in the district nursing service was high were also those districts with above average proportions of elderly in the population. (The relationship was significant at the 95% level using Spearman's rank correlation coefficient.) There are of course some exceptions. For example District 1 had a high proportion of its staff in the categories who mainly cared for the elderly but a below average proportion of elderly in the population. In contrast District 20 had the lowest proportion of staff (38%) in these categories but an above average proportion of elderly in its population.

Column c of Table 11.5 contains the district classification. The 24 health districts have been divided into six groups—suburban/growth areas, rural areas, resort/retirement areas, areas of traditional industry, service centres and new towns. These groups are based on a classification of local authority districts devised by Richard Webber and John Craig††. They used a wide range of social, economic and demographic characteristics of the districts, derived from census data, to group the districts into 30 relatively homogeneous clusters which they then combined into six 'families'. These correspond to our groups except that we have kept rural areas as a separate group from the resort/retirement area group and put the one central London district together with service centres.

There were few relationships between this classification of districts and the proportion of staff who worked mainly with the elderly. Not surprisingly the two districts in resort/retirement areas had the highest proportions of elderly in the population and were the two districts with

---

†The proportion of people aged 65 or more in the 24 health districts was 15.5%. The national average for 1980 was 15.1%. Population estimates were obtained from OPCS.

††See OPCS *Population Trends 5* HMSO Autumn 1976. The names assigned to some of the groups are self explanatory. 'Service centres' are large cities or important regional centres, typical examples of which are Nottingham, Southwark, Southampton and Wirral. Suburban and growth districts consist mainly of suburban and residential districts characterised by relatively large proportions of people in high socio-economic groups; typical examples are Stafford, Wycombe, Reigate and Barnet. Traditional industry areas are those industrial areas that are orientated to manufacturing and mining rather than services industries, for example Wakefield, Wolverhampton and Bolton. None of the districts mentioned here were included in the survey.

Table 11.4 Types of nurses employed in the district nursing service†—based on full-time equivalents of staff in post

Type of nurse	District																								All
	1	2*	3	4	5	6	7	8*	9	10	11*	12	13*	14	15*	16	17	18	19	20*	21	22	23	24	
	%	%	%	%	%	%	%	%	%	%	%	%	%	%	%	%	%	%	%	%	%	%	%	%	%
DN SRN +	47	37	35	43	57	32	44	42	40	40	47	46	62	31	45	41	60	41	40	38	46	40	37	49	43
DN SRN −	11	18	15	14	11	12	14	32	11	15	14	9	12	15	19	6	3	10	7	17	6	24	5	8	13
DN SEN +	4	12	15	9	10	18	7	4	22	14	14	5	23	10	—	10	12	26	15	9	10	14	28	15	13
DN SEN −	18	11	5	—	3	6	5	—	3	13	8	9	—	13	11	5	4	5	1	9	—	2	4	4	6
DN NR††	2	10	—	18	3	4	15	4	2	6	—	9	3	4	—	8	6	5	19	—	1	4	4	5	5
Aux	18	12	30	16	16	28	15	18	22	12	17	22	—	27	25	30	15	13	18	27	37	16	22	19	20
Number of nurses *(= 100%)*	90	67	81	44	115	111	80	56	110	82	72	64	65	95	91	40	67	39	100	47	138	101	95	145	1995

†The district nursing service includes district nurses and auxiliaries.

††DN NR denotes non-responding district nurses. Since the tables are based on staff in post it is necessary to include those who refused to be interviewed or who were not contacted. The non-responding district nurses are shown as a separate category because their qualifications were not known.

* denotes districts which have joint duty staff.

Table 11.5 The relationship between the proportion of staff working mainly with the elderly† and the proportion of elderly among the population

District and base (full-time equivalents)	Proportion of staff working mainly with the elderly†	District classification	Above average†† proportion of population aged 65+
a	b	c	d
6 (186)	58%	resort/retirement	√
5 (207)	53%	resort/retirement	√
1 (164)	52%	traditional industry	
23 (191)	51%	traditional industry	√
4 (106)	50%	service centre	√
10 (152)	50%	service centre	√
11 (170)	50%	suburban/growth	√
19 (176)	50%	traditional industry	
21 (293)	49%	service centre	√
2 (173)	47%	rural	
8 (132)	47%	rural	√
3 (173)	46%	service centre	√
16 (78)	46%	suburban/growth	
22 (210)	46%	traditional industry	
24 (296)	46%	suburban/growth	
13 (146)	45%	suburban/growth	
14 (213)	44%	traditional industry	
15 (219)	43%	rural	√
17 (152)	42%	service centre	
18 (93)	42%	suburban/growth	
7 (177)	41%	traditional industry	
9 (263)	41%	service centre	
12 (156)	39%	new town	
20 (111)	38%	traditional industry	√
All (4236) districts	47%		

†These staff comprised district nurses, auxiliaries, geriatric nurses and three quarters of the joint duty district nurse/midwives. The percentages are based on full-time equivalents of staff.
††The average proportion of the population aged 65+ was 15.5%.

nurses† with different attachment patterns for each of the 24 health districts in the survey. The top part of the table shows the proportions who were attached or not: the lower part the type of attachment worked by the attached nurses. As can be seen there was a wide variation between districts in the proportions of nurses who were attached to general practice—from 55% to 97% (Districts 3 and 17). The lower part of the table indicates a wide variation also in the type of attachment and patch working arrangements in existence in different health districts. The proportion of nurses who worked what can be called the full type of attachment, that is they covered all parts of A GP's area only, ranged from 14% to 79% (District 15 and 5).

The full type of attachment can be modified in two basic ways, firstly by dividing GP areas geographically so that nurses cover specific parts only, secondly by giving nurses geographical patches to cover in addition to the GP catchment area or the specific parts of it that they cover. Nurses whose attachments were modified in these ways fall into three groups as shown in the last three rows of Table 11.6, that is they worked a specific part of a GP area only, they worked in all parts but had an additional patch or they worked in a specific part of a GP area and had an additional patch. To look at the two modifications of attachment arrangements either the first and third or the second and third of these groups have to be added together to give the proportions who worked in a specific part of a GP area and the proportions who worked an additional patch.

Table 11.6 therefore shows that the proportion of nurses who were attached to specific parts of a GP area ranged from 11% (District 12) to 72% (District 15). The proportion who worked additional geographical patches varied from seven per cent to 67% (Districts 7 and 15).

Table 11.7 examines the relationship between the different types of attachment within districts. First the 24 districts are listed in descending order of the proportion of nurses who were attached to general practice in some way (column b). District 17 which had the highest rate of

†Including district nurses, midwives, joint duty staff, health visitors, auxiliaries and assistants and liaison nurses but excluding full-time relief nurses in these categories.

the highest proportions of staff concerned with their care. In addition, all but one of the suburban/growth districts had below average proportions of elderly and staff who worked mainly with the elderly.

11.2 Patterns of attachment to general practice

The different patterns of attachment and patch working identified by the survey were described in detail in Chapter 3, Table 3.4 showed these patterns for different types of nurses. Table 11.6 shows the proportions of

Table 11.6 Patterns of attachment and patch working in the 24 health districts

Working patterns	District 1	2	3	4	5	6	7	8	9	10	11	12	13	14	15	16	17	18	19	20	21	22	23	24	All
	%	%	%	%	%	%	%	%	%	%	%	%	%	%	%	%	%	%	%	%	%	%	%	%	%
Not attached	42	28	45	25	10	10	14	26	34	32	6	15	7	26	31	14	3	24	15	6	17	14	13	4	19
Attached	58	72	55	75	90	90	86	74	66	68	94	85	93	74	69	86	97	76	85	94	83	86	87	96	81
Number of nurses (= 100%)†	144	129	129	64	187	166	136	107	208	133	152	154	122	182	193	71	124	76	156	102	186	200	148	276	3545
	%	%	%	%	%	%	%	%	%	%	%	%	%	%	%	%	%	%	%	%	%	%	%	%	%
Attached and covers:																									
all parts of GP area	24	42	35	40	79	76	63	49	38	34	56	66	56	22	14	52	33	47	63	61	52	57	26	70	50
specific area only	14	12	29	33	12	13	30	19	18	13	14	9	32	25	19	30	33	16	18	11	28	20	13	20	21
all parts plus patch	28	22	20	16	8	8	2	28	29	25	25	23	11	22	14	9	15	21	14	23	13	20	28	9	17
specific areas plus patch	34	24	16	11	1	3	5	4	15	28	5	2	1	31	53	9	19	16	5	5	7	3	33	1	12
Number of attached nurses (= 100%)	84	92	72	48	168	149	117	79	137	90	143	131	113	136	134	61	120	58	133	96	155	183	129	266	2894

†The table includes those types of nurses who can be attached to general practice, that is district nurses, midwives, joint duty staff, health visitors and health visitor assistants, auxiliaries and liaison nurses. It however excludes full-time relief nurses in these categories.

attachment, 97%, is at the top of the list and District 3 which had the lowest rate, 55% is at the bottom. Seven of the 24 districts had attachment rates of 90% or more and a further seven had rates between 83% and 87%. Five districts had rates between 70% and 80% and the remaining five had attachment rates below 70%, the lowest being 55%.

There was no clear relationship between the type of district and the proportion of nurses in that district who were attached. However the three rural districts all had low attachment rates and the two resort/retirement districts had relatively high (90%) attachment rates. For all the other groups there was a wide variation in the attachment rates of districts within the same group. Suburban/growth districts tended to have higher levels of attachment—only one district, 18, had a lower than average proportion of attached nurses.

Table 11.6 showed that nationally among attached nurses 50% worked the full type of attachment and covered all parts of the GP's area. Thirty three per cent worked in specific parts of the GP's area and 29% worked in either all or specific parts of the catchment area but had a patch to cover in addition. The final three columns (d, e and f) of Table 11.7 use these national estimates of the prevalence of different types of attachment to show the relationship between patterns of attachment and patch working and the overall attachment rate shown in column b.

Column d therefore indicates those health districts where the proportion of attached nurses working in all parts of the GP area only was above the national estimate of 50%. As can be seen these are found exclusively in those districts where the overall attachment rate was above the average of 81%. Only two such districts had less than one half of their attached nurses working in all parts of GP areas. None of the districts with attachment rates below 80% had more than one half of their attached nurses working this full type of attachment.

The final two columns of Table 11.7 (e and f) show the districts with above average proportions working in specific parts of GP catchment areas and those with above average proportions of nurses working an additional patch. Both of these modifications of attachment working were found predominantly in health districts with low overall attachment rates.

All the rural districts and four out of the six service centre districts had above average proportions of nurses working an additional patch. Apart from this there was no relationship between the type of attachment operating in districts and the type of district.

In conclusion then those districts which had a high attachment rate also had above average proportions of attached nurses working full attachment schemes. Those districts with a lower attachment rate also had above average proportions of attached nurses working in specific parts of GP areas only and/or working patches in addition.

In Chapter 3 Table 3.4 showed that the proportion of nurses who were attached varied with the type of nurse. It might be expected, therefore, that within districts there would be variation in the attachment rates of different types of nurses. Table 11.8 shows the attachment rates for district nurses and health visitors. The districts were ordered by their overall attachment rate. Midwives, joint

Table 11.7 Patterns of attachment and patch working in health districts, by rate of attachment

District and base†		Proportion of nurses who were attached	District classification	Of attached nurses more than: ††		
				Half attached all parts only	A third worked in specific parts	A third had additional patch
a		b	c	d	e	f
17	(124)	97%	service centre		√	√
24	(276)	96%	suburban/growth	√		
11	(152)	94%	suburban/growth	√		
20	(102)	93%	traditional industry	√		
13	(122)	93%	suburban/growth	√		
5	(187)	90%	resort/retirement	√		
6	(166)	90%	resort/retirement	√		
23	(148)	87%	traditional industry		√	√
7	(136)	86%	traditional industry	√	√	
16	(71)	86%	suburban/growth	√	√	
22	(200)	86%	traditional industry	√		
12	(154)	85%	new town	√		
19	(156)	85%	traditional industry	√		
21	(186)	83%	service centre	√	√	
18	(76)	76%	suburban/growth			√
4	(64)	75%	service centre		√	
14	(182)	74%	traditional industry		√	√
8	(107)	74%	rural			√
2	(129)	72%	rural		√	√
15	(193)	69%	rural		√	√
10	(133)	68%	service centre		√	√
9	(208)	66%	service centre			√
1	(144)	58%	traditional industry		√	√
3	(129)	55%	service centre		√	√
All districts	(3545)	81%				

† The table includes those types of nurses who can be attached to general practice, that is district nurses, midwives, joint duty staff, health visitors, auxiliaries and liaison nurses. It however excludes full-time relief nurses in these categories.
†† The national estimates for these three groups were 50%, 33% and 29%. The words half and a third have been used on the table for simplicity. In the case of the final column the ticked districts are the same if 33% or 29% are used.

Table 11.8 Proportion of district nurses and health visitors who were attached, by district

Percentage attachment rate	District†																									All
	17	24	11	20	13	5	6	23	7	16	22	12	19	21	18	4	14	8	2	15	10	9	1	3		
All nurses††	97	96	94	94	93	90	90	87	86	86	86	85	85	83	76	75	74	74	72	69	68	66	58	55		81
District nurses	100	96	90	95	93	88	93	94	77	87	84	92	79	86	77	72	81	68	72	63	68	74	57	89		83
Health visitors	97	100	100	100	92	96	97	95	100	100	92	88	95	100	90	78	95	75	77	71	91	69	84	23		89

Number of nurses (base figures for the above proportions)

All nurses†† (= 100%)	124	276	152	102	122	187	166	148	136	71	200	154	156	186	76	64	182	107	129	193	133	208	144	129		3545
District nurses (= 100%)	52	112	62	37	57	86	76	64	45	31	95	50	68	72	26	29	62	40	47	67	71	68	68	56		1441
Health visitors (= 100%)	37	78	47	33	38	46	38	43	50	17	53	43	37	54	31	23	62	29	39	48	33	70	35	36		1020

†The districts are ordered from left to right by their overall attachment rate.
††The table includes those types of nurses who can be attached to general practice, that is district nurses, midwives, joint duty staff, health visitors, auxiliaries and liaison nurses. It however excludes full-time relief nurses in these categories.

duty staff and auxiliaries have been excluded since there were too few in individual districts to calculate rates.

Twelve of the districts had above average attachment rates for both district nurses and health visitors. These districts were obviously concentrated among those with high overall attachment rates. But among districts with low overall rates there was no consistent pattern. District 3, for instance, had a slightly higher than average proportion of attached district nurses (89%) and a low proportion of attached health visitors (23%). In contrast District 10 had a high proportion of attached health visitors (91%) and a low proportion of attached district nurses (68%).

11.3 Number of practices worked with

The number of practices which nurses worked with has been an important variable in previous chapters. Table 11.9 shows the number of practices which nurses worked with for each district. There was a great deal of variation between districts—the proportion working with only one practice, for instance, ranged from 23% (District 1) to 70% (District 11). All but one of the suburban/growth districts (Districts 11, 13, 16, 24) had high proportions of nurses working with only one practice. Apart from this there was no relationship between the number of practices worked with and the type of district. Districts with high attachment rates tended to have high proportions of nurses working with only one practice and the districts with below average attachment rates were those where higher proportions of nurses worked with large numbers of practices. This relationship between attachment and number of practices was discussed in Chapter 5.

Within districts there was variation between the different types of nurses in the number of practices worked with but, as for attachment, the pattern was different for each district.

A number of other variables which describe the way that nurses' work is organised—such as their daily work base and whether they have access to office space—were looked at for each district. There were wide variations between districts on all of these variables—in relation to daily work base, for instance, the proportion of nurses working from home varied from 61% (District 16) to 7% (Districts 4 and 10). There did not appear to be any relationship between these variables and the type of district, although these was a tendency for the

suburban/growth districts to have high proportions of nurses working from home and for service centre districts to have low proportions working from home. These patterns were not statistically significant and did not apply when the nurse types were considered separately. Neither did there appear to be any relationship between the length of nurses' experience and the type of district, although there was again a wide variation between districts.

11.4 Time spent travelling

As described in Section 6.4 the simplest method of grouping the way in which nurses spent their working time was to differentiate between time spent travelling, time spent on non-clinical activities and time spent with patients. This section looks at time spent travelling—its variation between districts and its relationship with type of district and attachment rate.

The breakdown of working time described above is shown for each of the districts, for district nurses, health visitors and auxiliaries, in Appendix Tables A11.1, A11.2 and A11.3. Tables 11.10 and 11.11 rank districts by the proportion of working time spent travelling and shown

Table 11.10 Proportion of time spent travelling by district nurses, by type of district and attachment rate.

District and base		Proportion of time spent travelling	District classification	Above average† proportion attached
a		b	c	d
12	(23)	28%	new town	√
3	(20)	26%	service centre	√
7	(22)	26%	traditional industry	
18	(17)	26%	suburban/growth	
21	(42)	26%	service centre	√
5	(47)	25%	resort/retirement	√
8	(20)	25%	rural	
9	(42)	25%	service centre	
11	(31)	25%	suburban/growth	√
13	(32)	25%	suburban/growth	√
14	(33)	25%	traditional industry	
19	(33)	25%	traditional industry	
2	(30)	24%	rural	
15	(39)	24%	rural	
16	(16)	24%	suburban/growth	√
20	(14)	24%	traditional industry	√
22	(59)	24%	traditional industry	√
23	(36)	24%	traditional industry	√
24	(52)	24%	suburban/growth	√
6	(36)	23%	resort/retirement	√
10	(26)	22%	service centre	
1	(32)	21%	traditional industry	
4	(7)	20%	service centre	
17	(27)	19%	service centre	√
All districts	(736)	24%		

†The average proportion of district nurses who were attached was 83%

Table 11.9 Number of practices worked with—by district

Number of practices	District																								
	1	2	3	4	5	6	7	8	9	10	11†	12	13	14	15	16†	17	18†	19	20	21	22	23	24†	All
	%	%	%	%	%	%	%	%	%	%	%	%	%	%	%	%	%	%	%	%	%	%	%	%	%
1	23	40	26	67	58	54	56	53	38	46	70	41	69	36	44	61	67	40	40	50	48	55	39	65	49
2	11	17	9	7	16	25	15	13	17	19	16	22	19	22	13	18	20	15	33	23	20	15	29	22	19
3 – 4	24	16	17	6	12	10	16	27	14	4	4	20	5	15	23	4	10	11	10	18	12	12	20	7	13
5+	36	24	24	19	7	9	9	6	27	19	10	13	5	13	20	15	3	29	14	7	14	17	5	4	14
No GP contact/ Don't know	6	3	24	1	7	2	4	1	4	12	–	4	2	14	*	2	*	5	3	2	6	1	7	1	5
Number of nurses†† (= 100%)	144	129	129	64	187	166	136	107	208	133	152	154	122	182	193	71	124	76	156	102	186	200	148	276	3545

†Denotes suburban/growth areas
††The table includes those types of nurses who can be attached to general practice, that is district nurses, midwives, joint duty staff, health visitors, auxiliaries and liaison nurses. It however excludes full-time relief nurses in these categories.

the type of district and attachment rate. Since few, if any, clear relationships emerged from our analysis of the data in the appendix tables, Tables 11.10 and 11.11 cover only the two main types of nurses—district nurses and health visitors.

Looking first at district nurses it can be seen that on average they spent 24% of their time travelling. The variation between districts was small, ranging from 19% (District 17) to 28% (District 12). It might have been expected that district nurses in rural districts spent a greater proportion of their time travelling than did staff in other types of districts. However the three rural districts were all on or just above the average. Each of the other types of districts were spread over the whole range of the proportions of time spent travelling.

Chapter 6 compared district nurses who were attached to general practice with those who were not and concluded that there were no differences between them in recorded travelling time. It was, therefore, not surprising to find no evidence of a relationship† between attachment rate and time spent travelling when the 24 districts were compared.

Table 11.11 relates to health visitors. Again the range of proportions of time spent travelling was small, from 13% in Districts 3, 4 and 10 to 20% in District 20. Also there was no relationship† between this and the attachment rate for health visitors. As with district nurses the rural districts were all on or just above the average. The service centres which are large cities or important regional centres tended to be clustered among those districts where health visitors spent a small proportion of their time travelling.

11.5 Time spent on non-clinical activities
To look at the way in which nurses spend their time other than travelling (which we have called activity time) time

---

†Relationships tested using Spearman's rank correlation coefficient

Table 11.11 Proportion of time spent travelling by health visitors, by type of district and attachment rate.

District and base		Proportion of time spent travelling	District classification	Above average† proportion attached
a		b	c	d
20	(33)	20%	traditional industry	√
13	(35)	19%	suburban/growth	√
16	(18)	19%	suburban/growth	√
22	(57)	19%	traditional industry	√
23	(38)	19%	traditional industry	√
8	(27)	18%	rural	
15	(42)	18%	rural	
7	(47)	17%	traditional industry	√
21	(53)	17%	service centre	√
2	(41)	16%	rural	
5	(41)	16%	resort/retirement	√
6	(31)	16%	resort/retirement	√
11	(45)	16%	suburban/growth	√
12	(36)	16%	new town	
14	(60)	16%	traditional industry	√
17	(37)	16%	service centre	√
18	(33)	16%	suburban/growth	√
24	(78)	16%	suburban/growth	√
1	(35)	15%	traditional industry	
9	(65)	14%	service centre	
19	(32)	14%	traditional industry	√
3	(34)	13%	service centre	
4	(20)	13%	service centre	
10	(29)	13%	service centre	√
All districts	(967)	16%		

†The average proportion of health visitors who were attached was 89%.

Table 11.12 Proportion of activity time spent on non-clinical activities by district nurses, by type of district

District and base		Proportion activity time on non-clinical	District classification	Above average† proportion worked from home	Above average†† proportion attached
a		b	c	d	e
4	(7)	42%	service centre		
21	(42)	42%	service centre	√	
10	(26)	41%	service centre		√
19	(33)	41%	traditional industry	√	
1	(32)	39%	traditional industry	√	
16	(16)	39%	suburban/growth	√	√
22	(59)	38%	traditional industry	√	√
23	(36)	38%	traditional industry	√	√
12	(23)	37%	new town	√	√
5	(47)	36%	resort/retirement		√
17	(27)	36%	service centre		√
20	(14)	36%	traditional industry	√	√
6	(36)	35%	resort/retirement		√
13	(32)	35%	suburban/growth	√	√
24	(52)	35%	suburban/growth		√
2	(30)	34%	rural	√	
7	(22)	34%	traditional industry		
9	(42)	33%	service centre		
11	(31)	31%	suburban/growth	√	√
18	(17)	31%	suburban/growth	√	
14	(33)	30%	traditional industry		
8	(20)	28%	rural	√	
3	(20)	27%	service centre		√
15	(39)	23%	rural		
All districts	(736)	35%			

†The average proportion of district nurses who worked from home was 61%.
††The average proportion of district nurses who were attached was 83%.

spent travelling is here excluded from the time recorded on the diaries. Activity time can then be divided into non-clinical time and time spent with patients and subsequently within those categories into fine detail. So far in the analysis described in this chapter we have not found a clear pattern of differences between different types of health districts. This suggests that it is not worth exploring the fine detail of activity time unless there are clear patterns emerging between districts in the proportion of time spent on non-clinical activity as opposed to time spent with patients. Again the full data for all districts are given in Appendix A11.4, A11.5 and A11.6.

Tables 11.12 and 11.13 show, for district nurses and health visitors, the proportion of activity time spent on non-clinical activities. Looking first at district nurses it can be seen that there was a large variation. Twenty three per cent of district nurse time in District 15 was spent on non-clinical activities compared with 42% in Districts 4 and 21. Again no clear pattern emerged between different types of health districts except that all the rural districts were in the lower part of the range, that is in districts where a below average proportion of activity time was spent on non-clinical work.

Columns d and e also show that there was no relationship between non-clinical activity and the proportion of district nurses who worked from home nor the proportion of district nurses who were attached to general practice.†

Health visitors spent more of their time on non-clinical activity than did district nurses. The proportions ranged from 49% to 63% (Districts 16 and 10). Clustered at the top of the range were five of the six service centres. Thus it appears that health visitors working in large cities spend

---

†Relationships tested using Spearman's rank correlation coefficient

Table 11.13 Proportion of activity time spent on non-clinical activities by health visitors, by type of district.

District and base a	Proportion of activity time on non-clinical b	District classification c	Above average proportion worked from clinics d	Above average†† proportion attached e
10 (29)	63%	service centre	√	√
3 (34)	60%	service centre		
21 (53)	60%	service centre	√	√
9 (65)	58%	service centre	√	
4 (20)	57%	service centre	√	
19 (32)	57%	traditional industry	√	√
8 (27)	56%	rural	√	
14 (60)	56%	traditional industry	√	√
24 (78)	56%	suburban/growth		√
5 (41)	55%	resort/retirement	√	√
13 (35)	55%	suburban/growth		√
18 (33)	55%	suburban/growth		√
11 (45)	54%	suburban/growth		√
12 (36)	54%	new town	√	
23 (38)	54%	traditional industry	√	√
1 (35)	53%	traditional industry		
20 (33)	52%	traditional industry		√
7 (47)	51%	traditional industry	√	√
15 (42)	51%	rural	√	
22 (57)	51%	traditional industry		√
2 (41)	50%	rural	√	
6 (31)	50%	resort/retirement		√
17 (37)	50%	service centre	√	√
16 (18)	49%	suburban/growth		√
All (967) districts	55%			

†The average proportion of health visitors based in clinics was 43%.
††The average proportion of health visitors who were attached was 89%.

more of their time on non-clinical activities than health visitors in other types of districts. This may be because they have a higher proportion of difficult cases and case conferences than health visitors in other districts. As Chapter 10 showed, most of these activities were accounted for by clerical and administrative work, telephone calls and meetings. As with district nurses, non-clinical time was not related to work base or attachment rate.

11.6 Groups of similar districts

In Section 11.1 we introduced a classification of districts based on a wide range of social and economic census variables which grouped the 24 health districts into six types. In the analyses which followed, the classification was used but the type of district seemed generally to have little bearing on variables such as attachment rate and time spent travelling. Before ending this chapter on differences between the districts, we shall look at the groups of districts to see what, if any, similarities exist within them.

Suburban/growth districts

Districts 11, 13, 16, 18 and 24 came into this category. For the present purpose the new town (District 12) has been included since there was only one new town in the sample and this was the category of districts to which it had most similarities.

Looking first at the data shown in Table 11.5 (proportion of staff who mainly cared for the elderly and proportion of elderly in the population) all but one of the districts had a less than average proportion of staff in this group. This reflects the relatively young demographic structure of suburban/growth districts. In all but one of the districts the attachment rate for the relevant nurses was 85% or

more—well above the average (Table 11.7). Four of the six districts were also similar in having an above average proportion of nurses who worked with one practice only (Table 11.9). Looking at the way in which district nurses spent their time (Tables 11.10, 11.12) there was no apparent similarity between these districts. This was not true however for health visitors. In these districts the proportion of time that health visitors spent travelling was average or above and the time spent on non-clinical work as opposed to contact with clients was average or below (Tables 11.11, 11.13).

Rural districts

Two of the rural districts were in Wales, the other in England (Districts 2, 8, 15). Two of the districts had higher than average proportions of elderly in the population but the proportion of staff who mainly cared for the elderly was either average or below (Table 11.5). All the rural districts had very similar attachment rates which were below the average for all districts (Table 11.7). They all employed joint duty district nurse/midwives. All districts were very similar in the proportions of time both district nurses and health visitors spent on travelling—they were either the average proportion or just above. On time spent on non-clinical work the district nurses in each of the three districts were below average. For health visitors the values ranged around the average and were very close together—50% to 56% (Tables 11.10—11.13).

Resort/retirement districts

Both resort/retirement districts (District 5 and 6) had high attachment rates of 90% and above average proportions of staff working with one general practice only (Tables 11.7, 11.9). They not surprisingly had the highest proportions of staff who mainly worked with the elderly (Table 11.5). For both district nurses and health visitors the proportions of time spent travelling and doing non-clinical work were very similar and very close to the averages for all districts (Tables 11.10—11.13).

Traditional industry districts

Seven districts, Districts 1, 7, 14, 19, 20, 22 and 23, fell into this category. On none of the variables discussed in this section was there any particular evidence of a similarity between districts. On all the key tables—Table 11.5, Table 11.7, Tables 11.10-11.13—traditional industry districts were scattered over most of the range of proportions.

Service centre districts

Like traditional industrial districts the group of service centre districts was large—Districts 3, 4, 9, 10, 17 and 21. Four of the districts had above average proportions of elderly in the population. These four had higher proportions of staff employed mainly in the care of the elderly than the other two. Thus there was no overall similarity among the districts. Two of the districts were in the North West region. Both these had above average attachment rates, the other four had below average rates. There were no similarities at all in the way in which district nurses spent their time. The opposite was the case for health visitors. In all but one of the districts health visitors spent average or below proportions of time travelling. In all but one they spent average or higher proportions of the rest of their time on non-clinical activities.

These last two types of district, traditional industry and service centre, account for almost one half of the districts in the survey. Fewer similarities emerged within them than within the other three groups discussed first—rural, resort/retirement and suburban/growth districts. This may be because the categories are too large and need to be sub-divided. However it is not clear how to sub-divide them—it could be done by demographic characteristics, socio-economic ones or on a regional basis. The choice is large and the possibilities we have explored have not identified groups that are any more homogenous than the larger categories.

Inner city districts

There are however four districts that in some sense form a group. They are derived from both traditional industry and service centre districts. They are districts which comprise parts of large conurbations in the North West, Midlands and London. They all are of low socio-economic status and are the four districts with the highest infant mortality rates among the districts in the survey. They are those which could be described as inner city districts—Districts 1, 3, 10 and 14.

These districts were not very similar demographically, two having above average and two below average proportions of elderly in the population. Not surprisingly, therefore, the proportions of staff who mainly worked with the elderly were not similar. However all the four districts had attachment rates well below the average and below average proportions of staff working with one general practice only. There was no similarity in the way in which district nurses divided their time but health visitors had patterns of work like those in service centre districts—that is they spent less time than average on travel and more time than average on non-clinical work as opposed to direct client contact.

The following tables provide a detailed breakdown of the working time of district nurses, health visitors and auxiliaries by district, as referred to in Sections 11.4 and 11.5. Tables A11.1, A11.2 and A11.3 show the proportions of working time spent on travel, non-clinical and patient-related activities in each district for the three types of nurses. Tables A11.4, A11.5 and A11.6 show the proportions of activity time spent on non-clinical, technical/nursing, advisory and unspecified activities in each district.

Table A11.1 Proportions of working time spent by district nurses on travel, non-clinical and patient-related activities

	District																								
---	1	2	3	4	5	6	7	8	9	10	11	12	13	14	15	16	17	18	19	20	21	22	23	24	All
	%	%	%	%	%	%	%	%	%	%	%	%	%	%	%	%	%	%	%	%	%	%	%	%	%
Travel Activities	21	24	26	20	25	23	26	25	25	22	25	28	25	25	24	24	19	26	25	24	26	24	24	24	24
non-clinical	31	25	20	34	27	27	25	21	25	32	23	27	27	23	17	29	29	23	31	27	31	29	29	26	26
with patients	46	47	50	46	46	49	46	52	48	46	50	45	47	51	58	46	50	43	46	42	45	46	48	48	48
unspecified	2	4	4	*	2	1	3	2	2	*	2	*	1	1	1	1	2	*	1	3	1	2	1	2	2
Average hours worked per week (= 100%)	30.7	35.1	39.8	36.5	32.7	46.4	37.7	30.1	36.1	33.2	36.5	32.5	36.1	36.9	34.4	33.5	35.8	27.2	31.7	30.4	37.4	22.7	33.1	28.6	33.6
Number of district nurses	32	30	20	7	47	36	22	20	42	26	31	23	32	33	39	16	27	17	33	14	42	59	36	52	736

Table A11.2 Proportions of working time spent by health visitors on travel, non-clinical and patient-related activities

	District																								
---	1	2	3	4	5	6	7	8	9	10	11	12	13	14	15	16	17	18	19	20	21	22	23	24	All
	%	%	%	%	%	%	%	%	%	%	%	%	%	%	%	%	%	%	%	%	%	%	%	%	%
Travel Activities	15	16	13	13	16	16	17	18	14	13	16	16	19	16	18	19	16	16	14	20	17	19	19	16	16
non-clinical	45	42	52	50	46	42	43	46	50	55	46	45	44	47	41	39	42	46	49	42	49	41	44	47	46
with patients	38	38	32	34	34	36	39	32	32	30	36	37	34	34	35	39	38	35	33	36	31	37	35	35	35
unspecified	2	4	3	3	4	6	2	4	4	2	3	2	2	3	6	2	4	3	4	2	3	3	2	2	3
Average hours worked per week (= 100%)	32.9	38.6	29.9	34.4	29.9	36.5	31.9	34.3	31.1	31.7	37.7	31.1	37.8	31.4	33.3	38.9	34.6	29.1	35.3	31.8	34.4	28.2	31.3	31.1	32.8
Number of health visitors	35	41	34	20	41	31	47	27	65	29	45	36	35	60	42	18	37	33	32	33	53	57	38	78	967

Table A11.3 Proportions of working time spent by auxiliaries on travel, non-clinical and patient-related activities

	District																								
---	1	2	3	4	5	6	7	8	9	10	11	12	13	14	15	16	17	18	19	20	21	22	23	24	All
	%	%	%	%	%	%	%	%	%	%	%	%	%	%	%	%	%	%	%	%	%	%	%	%	%
Travel Activities	28	23	18	25	31	19	20	23	15	25	23	22	–	11	19	24	18	22	22	17	23	28	15	25	21
non-clinical	14	11	32	11	14	19	26	12	21	16	14	21	–	19	9	13	11	13	18	12	18	13	10	12	16
with patients	58	65	45	62	54	60	52	65	62	58	63	57	–	69	71	63	71	65	58	70	57	61	75	61	62
unspecified	*	1	5	2	1	2	2	*	2	1	*	*	–	1	1	*	*	*	2	1	2	*	*	2	1
Average hours worked per week (= 100%)	17.7	22.3	30.7	37.6	22.4	27.9	27.1	17.1	25.7	28.8	20.7	15.1	–	28.7	23.9	15.9	22.3	17.3	35.6	28.8	34.5	20.5	24.9	20.8	24.6
Number of auxiliaries	21	16	25	6	34	31	9	18	38	9	25	22	–	25	36	16	17	11	18	13	46	29	33	43	541

Table A11.4 Proportions of activity time spent by district nurses on various activities

	District																								
	1	2	3	4	5	6	7	8	9	10	11	12	13	14	15	16	17	18	19	20	21	22	23	24	All
	%	%	%	%	%	%	%	%	%	%	%	%	%	%	%	%	%	%	%	%	%	%	%	%	%
Non-clinical	39	34	27	42	36	35	34	28	33	41	31	37	35	30	23	39	36	31	41	36	42	38	38	35	35
Technical and nursing	52	47	58	51	50	54	53	58	54	49	53	51	52	58	65	50	48	52	47	52	44	49	53	52	52
Advice	7	13	10	6	12	10	9	11	11	9	14	11	11	10	10	10	14	17	10	8	13	10	8	12	11
Unspecified	2	6	5	*	2	1	4	3	2	*	2	1	2	2	2	1	2	*	1	4	1	3	1	3	2
Average activity hours (= 100%)	*24.2*	*26.7*	*29.4*	*29.3*	*24.6*	*35.6*	*28.0*	*22.6*	*27.2*	*26.1*	*27.3*	*23.4*	*27.2*	*27.5*	*26.2*	*25.4*	*29.0*	*20.0*	*23.7*	*22.9*	*27.7*	*17.4*	*25.2*	*21.7*	*25.5*
Number of district nurses	32	30	20	7	47	36	22	20	42	26	31	23	32	33	39	16	27	17	33	14	42	59	36	52	736

Table A11.5 Proportions of activity time spent by health visitors on various activities

	District																								
	1	2	3	4	5	6	7	8	9	10	11	12	13	14	15	16	17	18	19	20	21	22	23	24	All
	%	%	%	%	%	%	%	%	%	%	%	%	%	%	%	%	%	%	%	%	%	%	%	%	%
Non-clinical	53	50	59	58	55	50	51	56	59	63	54	54	55	56	51	49	51	55	57	52	60	50	54	51	54
Technical and nursing	9	11	5	6	9	9	7	8	8	6	13	8	8	8	11	9	8	8	10	11	6	11	10	6	9
Advice	35	34	33	32	30	34	39	31	29	29	30	36	35	33	31	40	37	33	29	34	30	35	33	35	33
Unspecified	3	5	3	4	6	7	3	5	4	2	3	2	2	3	7	3	4	4	3	4	4	3	2	4	4
Average activity hours (= 100%)	*28.0*	*32.4*	*26.1*	*30.1*	*25.0*	*30.6*	*26.6*	*28.0*	*26.9*	*27.5*	*31.9*	*26.2*	*30.5*	*26.5*	*27.5*	*31.3*	*29.1*	*24.4*	*30.3*	*25.3*	*28.5*	*22.9*	*25.4*	*26.1*	*27.5*
Number of health visitors	35	41	34	20	41	31	47	27	65	29	45	36	35	60	42	18	37	33	32	33	53	57	38	78	967

Table A11.6 Proportions of activity time spent by auxiliaries on various activities

	District																								
	1	2	3	4	5	6	7	8	9	10	11	12	13	14	15	16	17	18	19	20	21	22	23	24	All
	%	%	%	%	%	%	%	%	%	%	%	%	%	%	%	%	%	%	%	%	%	%	%	%	%
Non-clinical	20	14	39	15	21	23	32	16	24	21	19	27	–	21	11	17	13	17	23	14	23	17	12	16	20
Technical and nursing	73	80	50	83	73	70	59	82	63	70	78	63	–	73	85	78	83	77	69	71	70	79	81	76	72
Advice	6	5	5	*	4	5	6	2	10	8	3	10	–	5	3	5	4	6	6	14	5	4	7	6	6
Unspecified	1	1	6	2	2	2	3	*	3	1	*	*	–	1	1	*	*	*	2	1	2	*	*	2	2
Average activity hours (= 100%)	*12.7*	*17.3*	*25.1*	*28.4*	*16.1*	*22.7*	*21.8*	*13.2*	*21.7*	*21.7*	*16.0*	*11.8*	*–*	*25.4*	*19.3*	*12.1*	*18.2*	*13.5*	*27.6*	*23.8*	*26.6*	*14.8*	*21.3*	*15.6*	*19.4*
Number of auxiliaries	21	16	25	6	34	31	9	18	38	9	25	22	–	25	36	16	17	11	18	13	46	29	33	43	541

12 Time spent with client groups in relation to the population

12.1 Rates and staffing ratios

The proportion of time which nurses spent with different client groups was described in Chapter 8. Using the same information from the diaries completed by nurses rates have been calculated to give the time spent with different client groups per head of the population in each particular potential client group. These rates have been calculated for each of the 24 health districts. It was only possible to do this for client groups defined by age and sex since information about the numbers of, for example, handicapped people, was not available by health district. Further details of how the rates were calculated are given in the appendix to the chapter.

Staffing ratios have also been calculated for each district using the numbers of relevant staff for each client group. The staff numbers were based on estimated full-time equivalents and adjusted to take account of non-response.

In Chapter 11 we saw that there was a wide variation between districts in the proportions of the different types of nurses they employed. This variation may be related to the population structure of the districts. Table 11.5, for instance, showed that, in general, the districts with a high ratio of staff who mainly cared for the elderly were those with a high proportion of people aged 65 or more in the population. This chapter considers the relationship between the rates representing the time spent with particular age and sex groups in a district and the relevant staffing ratios for the districts.

12.2 The elderly

The relevant staffing ratio for the elderly was based on district nurses, three quarters of the district nurse/midwives, auxiliaries and geriatric nurses because only these types of nurses spent a large proportion of their time with the elderly. Non-responding nurses—those who did not take part in the survey and those who did not complete a diary—were included. Thus the number of staff per 100,000 adults aged 65 or more was calculated for each district.

In Table 12.1, therefore, the districts are ranked according to this staffing ratio with the highest first (columns a and b). Column d contains the rate for adults aged 65 and over, that is, the number of hours per week spent per 100 adults aged 65 and over. Column c denotes those districts with a higher than average rate for those aged 65 and over and it is clear that it is the districts with high staffing ratios of staff who mainly care for the elderly which spend most time per head on the elderly.

12.3 Schoolchildren

Similarly Table 12.2 looks at the relationship between the

Table 12.1 Relationship between staffing ratio of staff who mainly work with the elderly and time spent on the elderly

District	Number of staff† per 100,000 adults aged 65 or more	Hours per week spent per 100 adults aged 65 or more by nurses working in the community	
a	b	Above average c	Rate d
4	608	✓	6.06
16	510	✓	4.66
1	489	✓	5.25
7	450		4.38
10	448	✓	4.73
3	435	✓	6.19
24	419	✓	5.24
19	356		4.09
18	339	✓	4.63
2	333	✓	4.62
21	325	✓	5.16
15	304	✓	5.38
22	285		3.89
13	284		4.07
23	283		4.25
12	269		3.34
14	254		4.15
20	248		3.64
17	231		3.65
11	225		3.72
9	222		3.77
8	220		3.39
5	218		3.32
6	213		3.94
All	392		4.40

†Includes district nurses, three quarters of district nurse/midwives, auxiliaries and geriatric nurses. Numbers are based on full-time equivalents and have been adjusted to take account of non-response.

school nursing staffing ratio and the time spent per head on schoolchildren. Again the districts are ranked by the staffing ratio, which is based on the number of school nurses and assistants per 100,000 children aged 5 to 15 (column b) and includes nurses who did not complete a diary. The number of hours per week spent per 100 children aged 5-16† is given in column d, and column c denotes those districts with a higher rate than the average. The districts with high school nursing staffing ratios are the districts which spend most time per head on schoolchildren.

12.4 Children aged less than five years old

Table 12.3 is more surprising. The districts are ranked by a staffing ratio, this time based on the number of health visitors and health visitor assistants per 100,000 children aged less than five years old. Again non-responding health visitors and assistants were included. Column d

†The diary age and sex codes used the grouping 5-16 whereas the population figures obtained grouped children aged 5-15. This should not affect comparison between districts however.

Table 12.2 Relationship between school nursing staffing ratio and time spent on schoolchildren

District	Number of nursing staff† per 100,000 children aged 5–15	Hours per week spent per 100 children aged 5–16†† by nurses working in the community	
a	b	Above average c	Rate d
4	182	√	1.50
21	127	√	1.78
3	92	√	1.21
10	92	√	1.21
23	73	√	1.28
2	71	√	1.21
7	70		0.83
18	66	√	1.39
22	66	√	1.21
1	55		0.83
9	55		0.87
14	50	√	0.90
19	50		0.79
15	49		0.84
5	43		0.74
16	40		0.22
24	37		0.78
17	33		0.57
11	27		0.79
8	24		0.56
6	20		0.88
13	20		0.34
20	12		0.37
12	11		0.46
All	52		0.89

†Includes school nurses and school nurse assistants. Numbers are based on full-time equivalents and have been adjusted to take account of non-response.

††The diary age and sex codes used the groupings 5–16 whereas the population figures grouped children aged 5–15. Comparison between districts should not be affected, however.

Table 12.3 Relationship between health visiting staffing ratio and time spent on children under five

District	Number of nursing staff† per 100,000 children aged under 5	Hours per week spent per 100 children aged under 5 by nurses working in the community	
a	b	Above average c	Rate d
6	525	√	3.79
10	503	√	3.32
12	464	√	3.39
16	459	√	4.33
13	455	√	3.32
15	424	√	3.95
5	415		2.78
8	400		3.05
18	392		2.96
3	391	√	3.92
1	383		2.94
11	373	√	3.25
23	364	√	3.41
24	357		2.79
9	352		3.28
14	340	√	3.40
20	336		2.74
21	332	√	3.44
19	325		2.51
17	314		2.87
22	309		2.73
2	282		2.72
7	265		2.88
4	194	√	3.54
All	362		3.15

†Includes health visitors and health visitor assistants. Numbers are based on full-time equivalents and have been adjusted to take account of non-response.

contains the rate for children under five and districts with above average rates are ticked in column c. The clear relationship† between high staffing ratios and high rates which was apparent in the previous two tables is not present in Table 12.3. The districts which spent most time per head on children less than five are not, in general, the districts with the highest health visiting staffing ratios. Indeed the district with the lowest staffing ratio, District 4, has a rate of 3.54, well above the average. This lack of relationship is surprising because health visitors have a clearly defined role in relation to a specific client group, the under fives, perhaps more so than many other types of nurses working in the community.

12.5 Women aged 16-44

The rates for women aged 16-44 were looked at in relation to a staffing ratio based on midwives and district nurse/midwives but there was no relationship between them.

The elderly, women in the reproductive age group, the under fives and schoolchildren are age and sex groups where it is clear which particular types of nurses working in the community serve their needs. It is less appropriate to examine staffing ratios and rates for other age and sex

†Relationships were tested for statistical significance using Spearman's rank correlation coefficient.

groups as it is not clear on which types of nurses the staffing ratios should be based.

12.6 Variations between districts

Apart from considering the relationships between hours spent per week per head of various client groups and the relevant staffing ratios, the tables show the generally very wide variation between districts in the level of provision of different kinds of community nursing. Table 12.1 shows for example that staffing ratios of staff who mainly care for the elderly varied from 213 per 100,000 adults aged 65 or more to 608 (Districts 6 and 4). District 4 was the district which employed a large number of specialist geriatric nurses. Staffing ratios of health visiting staff varied to a similar degree and strangely the same two districts were at the extremes. For health visiting District 4 had the lowest staff ratio (194) and District 6 the highest (525). They both however had very similar rates of hours per week spent per 100 children under five. District 4 also had the highest ratio of school nursing staff, 182 per 100,000 children aged 5-15. This ratio varied more than those for health visiting or care of the elderly, the lowest ratio being only 11 per 100,000 (District 12).

In general these large differences between districts in staffing ratios resulted in smaller differences between the hours spent per head of the population. For example for health visiting the rate varied from 3.32 to 6.06, for care of the elderly from 2.51 to 4.33. Whilst large they are not as great as the almost threefold differences in the staffing ratios.

Appendix to Chapter 12

A12.1 Method of calculating the rates

Chapter 8 described the way that nurses recorded details of the patients they saw and the clinics they carried out. In particular they recorded the age and sex of the patients they spent time with. (See Chapter 8 for a list of the age and sex groups used.) This means that all the periods of time (except for time in clinics) which a nurse spent with patients of any particular age and sex group can be added together to give a total time†, excluding time in clinics, which the nurse spent with patients of that age and sex group during her week of diary recording. The totals for all of the nurses working in a health district were then added together to give the total time, excluding clinics, spent on patients of that age and sex group by the community nursing staff of the district.

Similarly the total time† spent on a particular kind of clinic by a district's community nursing staff during one week was calculated. Most kinds of clinics concentrate on the particular age and sex group, for instance, time spent doing ante-natal and post-natal clinics is spent with women aged 16–44. Thus the time spent on each kind of clinic was added to the total time spent with the appropriate age and sex group to provide *an overall total of all time, including time in clinics, spent with patients of each age and sex group in each district.* Table A12.1 lists the different kinds of clinics and the age and sex groups to which the time spent on each clinic was added.

Information on the age and sex distribution of the population of each sampled health district was obtained†† and the number of people in each of the age and sex groups used in the survey was calculated. The proportions of the population found in the different age and sex groups are shown for each district in Table A12.2.

For each district the total time spent on a particular age and sex group was then divided by the size of that age and sex group to give time spent per week per 100 people in that age and sex group for that district. The rates for all age and sex groups in each district are given in Table A12.3. The rates for all 24 districts combined are shown in Table A12.4.

The rates shown in column c were based on the nurses who completed the diary. The time spent on the different age and sex groups by nurses who did not take part in the survey at all and by nurses who were interviewed but did

---

†As in previous chapters this only includes time spent on technical, nursing, advisory and unspecified activities with patients. Non-clinical and travel time are excluded.
††Population distributions for health districts were obtained from Population Statistics Division 2 of OPCS.

Table A12.1 Age and sex groups to which time spent in clinics was added.

Clinic	Age and sex group time added to
1 Ante-natal and post-natal	Women 16–44
2 Well baby, infant welfare, child health	Children 5–15 for school nurses and assistants Children < 5 for all other types of nurses
3 Development assessment	Children 5–15 for school nurses and assistants Children < 5 for all other types of nurses
4 Immunisation and vaccination	Children 5–15
5 Rubella vaccination	Children 5–15
6 Mothercraft/parentcraft	Women 16–44
7 Family planning	Women 16–44
8 Well woman, cytology	Women 16–44
9 Hearing and vision	Children 5–15
10 School medicals/hygiene	Children 5–15
11 Health education	Children 5–15
12 GP surgery session	omitted†
13 Other	distributed amongst the age and sex groups in the same proportions as the rest of time spent on clinics.

---

†As GP surgery sessions are likely to cover most age and sex groups no attempt was made to assign this time to any particular group or to apportion the time. Only GP employed nurses spent substantial amounts of time on GP surgery sessions so the omission does not affect the rates for other types of nurses.

not complete a diary could not be included. However as was shown in Chapter 1 response to the survey varied between districts and types of nurse therefore it was felt to be more accurate to weight the rates by adding the estimated amount of time spent on patients by non-responding nurses. These extra amounts of time have been estimated using information provided by those nurses who did complete the diaries. The adjusted rates as shown in column d of Table A12.4 of course make the assumption that nurses who did not complete the diary had similar patterns of work to those who did complete the diary.

For each district the rate for children less than five was weighted to take account of the non-response of health visitors and health visitor assistants in that district because most of the total time spent on these children was attributable to those types of nurses. Similarly the rate for children aged 5–15 was weighted to take account of the non-response of school nurses and school nurse assistants in each district. The non-response of midwives was used to weight the rates for women aged 16–44.

The same weight was applied to all four rates relating to men and women aged 65 and over—the weight was based on the non-response of district nurses, auxiliaries and geriatric nurses in each district. For the three remaining age and sex groups—men aged 16–44 and women and men aged 45–64—the rates were low and there were no particular types of nurses who spent a large amount or proportion of their time on these groups. In fact all types of nurses spent small proportions of time on them. The same weight was applied to the rates for all three groups and for all districts. This weight was based on the overall non-response less the non-response already accounted for.

The total time spent on all patients was weighted by the overall non-response. The total times spent on children less than five, children aged 5–15, women aged 16–44 and men and women aged 65+ were weighted by the non-response of the appropriate types of nurses. These totals were then subtracted from the first overall total to leave total time spent on men 16–44 and men and women 45–64, but adjusted for non-response. This total was then divided by the actual time spent on these three groups to provide the weight for non-response.

It was originally intended to carry out this calculation for each district but the first few calculations found that the resulting weights were small and did not vary a great deal between district so the overall weight was used to cover all districts.

The non-response adjusted rates for all age and sex groups in each district are given in the appendix in Table A12.5.

A12.2 Rates for different age and sex groups
Table A12.4 shows that much more time was spent per head on women and men aged 75 and over than on any of the other groups. Because people aged 75 and over are a relatively small proportion of the population this shows up more clearly in the comparison of rates than it did in the comparison of proportions of time spent on different age and sex groups in Table 8.5. Women and men aged 65–74 and children less than five also had high rates. Men tended to have lower rates than women of the same age group—Table 8.5 showed a lower proportion of time was spent on the men in each age group and adjusting for the population distribution would obviously have little effect on that particular comparison. Men aged 16–44, as expected, had the lowest rate.

A12.3 Adjustments for non-response
In Tables 12.1, 12.2 and 12.3 both the staffing ratios and the rates used have been weighted to allow for non-response. When we first investigated the relationships between staffing ratios we drew up these tables in three

Table A12.4 Hours per week spent per 100 of each age and sex group in all districts

	a	b	c	d
Age and sex group	Population (hundreds)	Basic rate		Rate adjusted for non-response
Children < 5	(3157)	2.78		3.15
Children 5–15	(7906)	0.80		0.89
Women 16–44	(10875)	0.86		1.08
Men 16–44	(11157)	0.09		0.10
Women 45–64	(6158)	0.70		0.76
Men 45–64	(5829)	0.35		0.38
Women 65–74	(2925)	2.46		2.97
Men 65–74	(2199)	1.76		2.13
Women 75+	(2184)	6.38		7.70
Men 75+	(986)	5.25		6.34

Table A12.2 Age and sex distribution of the population in each sampled health district†

Age & sex group	District																								
	1	2	3	4	5	6	7	8	9	10	11	12	13	14	15	16	17	18	19	20	21	22	23	24	All
	%	%	%	%	%	%	%	%	%	%	%	%	%	%	%	%	%	%	%	%	%	%	%	%	%
Children < 5	6.3	6.6	5.8	4.5	5.3	4.5	7.4	5.3	5.9	5.0	5.4	5.8	6.0	6.2	6.0	6.5	6.0	6.8	5.9	6.0	5.5	6.4	5.4	6.6	5.9
Children 5–14	15.8	16.4	14.4	9.3	13.2	12.3	16.1	13.4	15.6	12.4	14.2	15.0	14.9	15.8	14.6	17.1	15.3	18.2	15.4	15.2	13.7	14.8	15.1	16.0	14.8
Women 15–44	21.0	20.6	19.4	26.9	18.9	17.5	21.9	18.4	20.1	22.9	21.1	21.4	20.6	18.9	18.9	18.8	21.3	21.9	20.4	20.1	20.2	20.7	19.8	20.7	20.4
Men 15–44	21.3	21.2	19.0	21.3	19.3	17.2	22.5	22.2	19.9	21.6	19.9	22.1	23.4	19.5	20.5	23.1	21.9	21.7	21.3	19.5	21.4	21.5	20.0	20.9	
Women 45–64	10.9	10.7	12.1	11.8	11.9	12.5	10.2	11.8	11.9	11.8	11.9	11.5	10.9	12.4	11.8	11.4	11.1	10.3	11.6	11.7	12.1	11.4	11.6	11.0	11.5
Men 45–64	10.8	10.7	12.0	9.9	10.1	9.9	10.8	10.6	11.4	10.6	10.7	11.4	10.6	12.2	10.7	11.3	11.0	10.1	10.9	10.7	10.9	11.2	11.5	11.0	10.9
Women 65–74	5.1	5.0	5.9	6.0	7.4	9.1	3.8	6.3	5.4	5.8	6.0	4.4	4.7	5.4	6.3	4.3	4.8	4.1	5.1	5.7	5.9	4.8	6.0	4.2	5.5
Men 65–74	3.7	3.9	4.6	3.9	5.2	5.5	3.3	4.7	4.1	4.1	4.6	3.7	3.8	4.1	4.3	3.5	3.7	3.1	3.9	4.3	4.1	3.9	4.6	3.5	4.1
Women 75+	3.5	3.3	4.7	4.8	6.2	8.3	2.5	4.7	4.1	4.1	4.4	3.1	3.2	3.8	4.9	2.9	3.2	2.5	3.9	4.6	4.4	3.5	4.1	3.1	4.1
Men 75+	1.4	1.5	2.1	1.6	2.6	3.2	1.5	2.3	1.9	1.6	1.9	1.5	1.9	1.7	2.2	1.1	1.6	1.4	1.5	2.3	1.8	1.7	2.0	1.5	1.8
Population†† (= 100%)	1787	2147	1442	1069	2809	2308	2689	1879	3576	1857	2318	2496	1970	3048	2267	840	2387	1084	2466	1673	2873	2686	2251	3456	53376

†Population figures were obtained from Population Statistics Division of OPCS.
††Each of these figures should be multiplied by 100.

Table A12.3 Rates indicating hours spent per 100 on each age and sex group in each district—based on nurses who completed the diary only

Age & sex group	District																							
	1	2	3	4	5	6	7	8	9	10	11	12	13	14	15	16	17	18	19	20	21	22	23	24
Children < 5	2.58	2.72	3.65	2.95	2.22	2.89	2.55	2.44	2.90	2.45	3.11	2.69	2.70	3.14	3.32	4.11	2.60	2.96	2.01	2.61	3.27	2.55	3.01	2.61
Children 5–15	0.80	1.17	1.15	1.33	0.51	0.80	0.73	0.37	0.79	0.98	0.79	0.46	0.34	0.79	0.72	0.19	0.52	1.39	0.79	0.37	1.60	0.98	1.04	0.71
Women 16–44	0.58	1.02	1.03	0.48	0.70	0.75	0.85	0.72	0.98	0.67	0.77	0.92	1.14	0.82	0.98	1.01	0.73	0.68	1.13	0.72	1.04	0.74	0.87	0.99
Men 16–44	0.11	0.14	0.05	0.04	0.08	0.14	0.03	0.06	0.10	0.12	0.13	0.05	0.05	0.08	0.15	0.05	0.05	0.08	0.05	0.03	0.12	0.18	0.08	0.08
Women 45–64	0.73	0.92	0.69	0.41	0.52	0.76	0.40	0.68	0.56	0.81	1.02	0.43	0.68	0.47	1.00	1.48	0.85	0.90	0.64	0.41	0.82	0.51	0.89	0.77
Men 45–64	0.42	0.60	0.41	0.36	0.28	0.29	0.19	0.18	0.38	0.41	0.41	0.18	0.31	0.33	0.62	0.46	0.30	0.30	0.39	0.27	0.34	0.35	0.41	0.33
Women 65–74	2.71	2.95	3.33	2.51	1.70	2.29	1.53	1.65	2.63	2.18	2.27	1.93	1.83	2.16	3.63	4.31	2.26	4.43	2.37	1.42	3.24	2.79	2.52	2.77
Men 65–74	2.54	2.04	2.34	1.32	1.09	1.52	0.54	1.09	2.23	1.77	1.70	1.11	1.72	1.89	2.92	3.60	1.94	2.56	1.79	1.15	2.02	1.75	1.88	1.66
Women 75+	6.70	6.54	8.39	5.92	5.31	5.29	6.75	5.50	4.54	5.30	6.53	4.65	7.29	5.93	8.82	10.30	6.17	6.86	5.65	4.94	9.17	6.19	6.96	8.32
Men 75+	5.57	8.16	4.71	4.19	4.50	4.89	3.17	4.68	6.18	3.22	6.02	3.37	5.89	5.54	6.92	11.34	3.97	4.31	3.80	4.93	5.00	5.13	7.14	5.87

different ways—without adjusting for non-response on either the rates or staffing ratios, adjusting the rates but not the staffing ratios and adjusting both figures as in the tables shown. The three methods produced very similar tables, making only minor differences in the ranking by staffing ratios and in the relative rates. Adjusting for non-response did not, therefore, appear to introduce any bias and we decided to use the adjusted rates and ratios as they should provide a more accurate representation of a district's work and staffing.

Table A12.5 Rates indicating hours spent per 100 on each age and sex group in each district—weighted to take into account non-response

Age & sex group	District																							
	1	2	3	4	5	6	7	8	9	10	11	12	13	14	15	16	17	18	19	20	21	22	23	24
Children < 5	2.94	2.72	3.92	3.54	2.78	3.79	2.88	3.05	3.28	3.32	3.25	3.39	3.32	3.40	3.95	4.33	2.87	2.96	2.51	2.74	3.44	2.73	3.41	2.79
Children 5–15	0.83	1.21	1.21	1.50	0.74	0.88	0.83	0.56	0.87	1.21	0.79	0.46	0.34	0.90	0.84	0.22	0.57	1.39	0.79	0.37	1.78	1.21	1.28	0.78
Women 16–44	0.92	1.43	1.03	0.80	0.85	0.75	1.06	0.81	1.19	0.84	0.77	1.23	1.52	1.28	0.98	1.19	1.07	1.02	1.28	0.81	1.43	0.86	1.13	1.16
Men 16–44	0.12	0.15	0.05	0.04	0.09	0.15	0.03	0.07	0.11	0.13	0.14	0.05	0.05	0.09	0.16	0.05	0.05	0.09	0.05	0.03	0.13	0.20	0.09	0.09
Women 45–64	0.80	1.00	0.75	0.45	0.57	0.83	0.44	0.74	0.61	0.88	1.11	0.47	0.74	0.51	1.09	1.61	0.93	0.98	0.70	0.45	0.89	0.56	0.97	0.84
Men 45–64	0.46	0.65	0.45	0.39	0.31	0.32	0.21	0.20	0.41	0.45	0.45	0.20	0.34	0.36	0.68	0.50	0.33	0.33	0.43	0.29	0.37	0.38	0.45	0.36
Women 65–74	3.58	3.30	4.47	4.50	1.93	2.65	2.56	1.93	2.86	3.43	2.32	2.55	2.03	2.61	3.69	4.99	2.48	4.63	2.99	1.86	3.54	2.96	2.68	3.43
Men 65–74	3.36	2.28	3.14	2.37	1.23	1.76	0.90	1.27	2.43	2.78	1.74	1.47	1.91	2.28	2.97	4.16	2.13	2.67	2.26	1.51	2.20	1.86	2.00	2.06
Women 75+	8.86	7.31	11.27	10.62	6.02	6.11	11.29	6.43	4.94	8.33	6.68	6.15	8.09	7.17	8.97	11.92	6.79	7.16	7.13	6.47	10.01	6.57	7.41	10.31
Men 75+	7.36	9.14	6.33	7.52	5.10	5.65	5.30	5.47	6.73	5.06	6.16	4.46	6.53	6.70	7.04	13.12	4.36	4.50	4.80	6.46	5.46	5.45	7.60	7.28

Appendix: Questionnaire and diary

S 1141   SURVEY OF COMMUNITY NURSES

Interviewer Name ....

Authorisation No ....

Time interview started ....

SERIAL
NUMBER   District /Sector   Informant

DATE OF
INTERVIEW   Day   Month

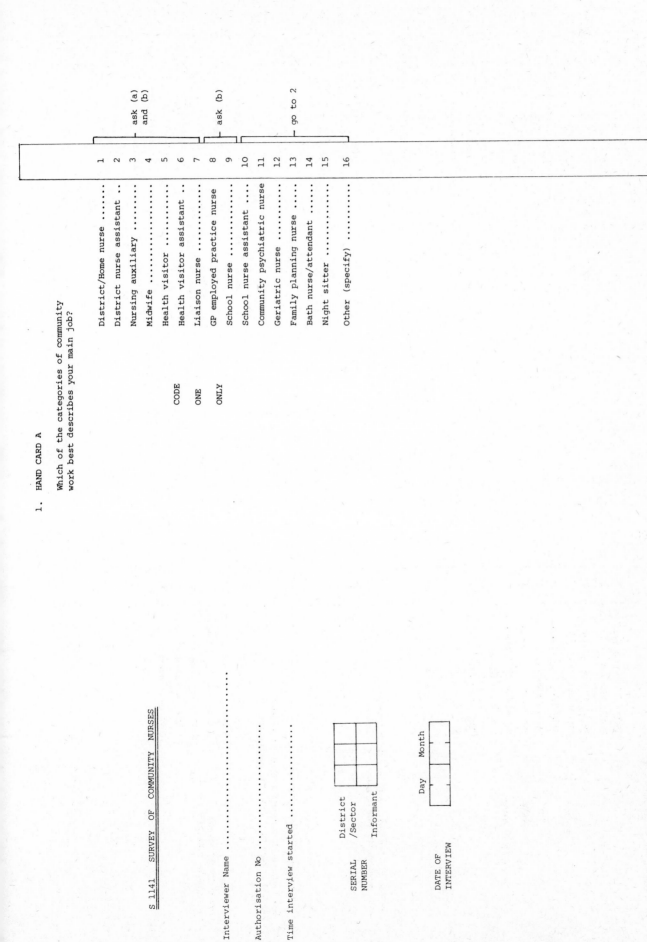

1. HAND CARD A

Which of the categories of community
work best describes your main job?

CODE   District/Home nurse   1
            District nurse assistant ..   2
ONE   Nursing auxiliary   3   ask (a)
            Midwife   4   and (b)
ONLY   Health visitor   5
            Health visitor assistant ..   6
            Liaison nurse   7
            GP employed practice nurse   8   ask (b)
            School nurse   9
            School nurse assistant   10
            Community psychiatric nurse   11
            Geriatric nurse   12
            Family planning nurse   13   go to 2
            Bath nurse/attendant   14
            Night sitter   15
            Other (specify)   16

-3-

2. (continued)

(a) HAND CARD B

Do you have any special responsibility for any of these services?

	CODE	School health	1
	ALL	Family planning	2
	THAT	Psychiatry	3
	APPLY	Geriatrics	4
		Hospitals	5
		Paediatrics	6
		Stoma Care	7
		Mental/Physical handicap	8
		T.B./Chest diseases	9
		Other (specify)	10
		None	11

(b) Apart from your main job, do you do any sessions in family planning clinics?

| Yes | 1 |
| No | 2 |

2. How many years altogether have you worked as a (FROM Q1) in the community?

Less than 1 year	1
1 but less than 5 years	2
5 but less than 10 years	3
10 but less than 15 years	4
15 but less than 20 years	5
20 years or more	6

ADD TOGETHER BROKEN PERIODS OF SERVICE

3. Have you had any other experience in the community at any level?

| Yes | 1 | ask (a) & (b) |
| No | 2 | go to 4 |

(a) HAND CARD A - What was that job?

	CODE	District/Home nurse	1
	ALL	District nurse assistant	2
	THAT	Nursing auxiliary	3
	APPLY	Midwife	4
		Health visitor	5
		Health visitor assistant	6
		Liaison nurse	7
		GP employed practice nurse	8
		School nurse	9
		School nurse assistant	10
		Community psychiatric nurse	11
		Geriatric nurse	12
		Family planning nurse	13
		Bath nurse/attendant	14
		Night sitter	15
		Other (specify)	16

(b) How many years altogether did you work as a (FROM Q3a) ?

Less than 1 year	1
1 but less than 5 years	2
5 but less than 10 years	3
10 but less than 15 years	4
15 but less than 20 years	5
20 years or more	6

ADD TOGETHER BROKEN PERIODS OF SERVICE AND DIFFERENT TYPES OF SERVICE

4.

Apart from your main work as (FROM Q1) do you do any relief work?

Yes	1	ask (a) & (b)
No	2	go to 5
Full-time relief nurse	3	go to 5

(a) May I just check - do you do covering or relief work:-

RUNNING PROMPT: as part of formal arrangements with specific GPs, Clinics, or other community nursing staff or informally for colleagues? ....

Specific	1
	2

(b) Thinking about the last month, what proportion of your working and on call time was spent doing relief work?

Less than ¼	1
¼ but less than ½ ...	2
½ but less than ¾ ...	3
¾ but less than total	4
Total	5

DNA CODE 8 AT Q1	Y	go to 8
DNA CODES 9-16 AT Q1	X	go to 11

5.

I'd now like to read a definition to you -

"Attachment or alignment are formal arrangements under which staff are responsible for providing services to people on the lists of specified general practitioners".

(Apart from any relief work) Are you attached or aligned to general practitioners in this way at all?

Yes	1	go to 6
No	2	ask (a)

(a) May I just check - Does that mean you work a geographical patch only?

Yes	1	go to 8
No	2	ask (b)

(b) So you are neither formally attached or aligned and you do not work entirely on a geographical patch system, how then is your work organised?

PROBE FULLY

6.

Do you care for patients in all parts of the GP's catchment area or only those who live in specific areas?

All parts	1
Specific areas	2

7.

Do you care only for people on specific GP lists, or are you responsible for an additional geographical patch?

Specific GP lists only	1
Specific GP lists plus patch	2

8.

How many GPs do you work with?

One	1	go to 9
Two	2	
Three	3	
Four to six .	4	ask (a)
Seven to ten	5	
More than ten	6	

(a) Are they all (both) in the same practice?

Yes	1	go to 9
No	2	ask (b)
Don't know	3	go to 9

(b) How many practices are involved?

Two	1
Three	2
Four	3
More than four	4
Don't know ...	5

9.

Are the general practitioners (is the general practitioner) working in a health centre or in their (his) own practice premises?

Health centre	1
Own practice premises	2
Both health centre and practice premises	3
Don't know	4

10. On average on how many working days per week do you have contact, either in the form of personal discussions or over the telephone, with any of your clients'/patients' GPs? On:-

RUNNING PROMPT

Less than one day a week	1
One day	2
Two days	3
Three days	4
Four days	5
Five days or more?	6

11. In your opinion are there are particular groups of clients/patients in your district that are in need of more care from nurses working in the community?

HAND CARD C

CODE ALL THAT APPLY

Pregnant women	1
Mothers and new babies	2
Under 5's	3
School children	4
One parent families	5
Elderly living alone	6
Elderly (generally)	7
Mentally handicapped	8
Physically handicapped	9
Mentally ill	10
Terminally ill	11
Post-operative/Hospital discharges	12
Ethnic minorities	13
Relatives of clients/patients	14
Other (specify)	15
None	16 go to 12

ask (a)

IF MENTIONED MORE THAN ONE GROUP

(a) Which group, of those you have mentioned, do you think is most in need of more care from nurses working in the community?

ENTER CODE FROM ABOVE [ ]

12. Do you do any 'on call' duty?

Yes	1	ask (a)
No	2	go to 13

(a) On average, for how many hours a week are you 'on call'?

HOURS PER WEEK [ ]

Unable to give an average (Specify on call arrangements)   0

13. (Excluding 'on call' time) How many hours on average do you work in a week?

HOURS PER WEEK [ ]

14. (Excluding 'on call' days) On how many days (nights) a week do you normally work?

DAYS PER WEEK [ ]

15. When you make visits either to clients/patients or other places as part of your work, how do you normally travel?

PROMPT AS NECESSARY

CODE ONE ONLY

DNA no visits ..	1 go to 17
Car	2
Public transport	3
On foot	4
Bicycle	5
Motorbike/Moped	6
Other	7 go to 16

16. How do you feel about the amount of travelling involved in your job? Is it:-

RUNNING PROMPT

far too much	1
too much	2
or is it about right?	3
(SPONTANEOUS ONLY) too little	4

-9-

84

17. Where do you work from on a daily basis?

PROMPT AS NECESSARY

CODE
ONE
ONLY

Home	1
Clinic	2
Health centre	3
Practice premises	4
Hospital	5
Community health office	6
School	7
Other (specify)	8

go to 19

go to 18

18. Do you have:-

RUNNING
PROMPT

your own office ...	1
shared office space	2
or no office?	3

19. DNA NURSING AUXILIARY, BATH NURSE (CODES 3,14 AT Q1) X   go to 25
    DNA NIGHT SITTER (CODE 15 AT Q1) Y   go to 22

Do you have any access to a treatment or interview room where you can see clients/patients in private?

Yes, access to treatment and/or interview room	1
No access to either treatment or interview room	2
DNA only do home visits	3
Other (specify)	4

20. DNA NURSE ASSISTING A SERVICE (CODES 2,6,10 AT Q1) X   go to 22
    DNA FULL TIME RELIEF NURSE (CODE 3 AT Q4) Y

Excluding relief work, do you have any staff that you personally can call on for assistance with clinical work?

(EXCLUDE INFORMAL ARRANGEMENTS WITH FRIENDS)

Yes	1	ask (a)
No	2	go to 21

(a) What kinds of staff assist you?

CODE
ALL
THAT
APPLY

District nurse assistant	1
Health visitor assistant	2
Nursing auxiliary	3
Bath nurse/assistant ...	4
Pupil or student nurse .	5
Other (specify)	6

21. Do you have any staff you can call on for assistance with clerical work?

Yes	1
No	2

22. What nursing qualifications do you have?

HAND CARD D

SRN or RGN	State registered nurse or Registered general nurse	1
SEN	State enrolled nurse	2
RMN	Registered mental nurse	3
SCM or CMB	part 1 State certified midwife or Certified midwives board	4
RSCN or RFN	Registered sick childrens nurse or Registered fever nurse	5
CODE HV Cert	Health Visitors Certificate	6
ALL NDN Cert or SEN Cert in DN	District nursing Certificates	7
THAT QIDN	Queens Institute of district nursing	8
APPLY BTA Cert	Thoracic nursing Certificate	9
	Obstetrics Certificate	10
	Orthopaedics Certificate	11
	Family Planning Certificate/Diploma	12
	Health Education Certificate	13
	Other (specify)	14
	None	15 go to 23

23. HAND CARD E

Do you have a teaching instructors or tutors certificate or any other job related qualifications?

CODE	Health Visitor Tutor	1
ALL	District Nurse Tutor	2
THAT	Midwifery Teachers Certificate	3
APPLY	Practical Work Teachers Certificate	4
	Field Work Certificate	5
	Instructing Nurse	6
	Community Health Nurse Certificate	7
	Other (specify)	8
	None	9 go to 24

24. Have you been on any management courses since starting your current job?

Yes ... 1

No ... 2

25. Have you been on any refresher courses or done any in-service training for your current job?

HAND CARD F

Refresher courses	1
Health education	2
Parentcraft/Mothercraft	3
Audiometry, audio visual screening	4
Study days on specific conditions	5
Red Cross proficiency certificate	6
General or community nursing	7
On the job training	8
Other courses (specify)	9
None	10

27. If you had more time, would you like to do more counselling and health education?

Yes	1	ask (a)
No	2	go to 28

(a) Which particular area would you like to spend more time on?

HAND CARD G

Pregnancy and labour	1
Nutrition incl. infant feeding	2
Child care/child development/parentcraft	3
Immunisation and vaccination	4
Family planning incl. sterilisation	5
Marital and psychosexual problems	6
Physical health problems	7
Mental health problems	8
Health education in schools	9
Other (specify)	10

CODE ALL THAT APPLY

ENTER CODE FROM ABOVE

IF MENTIONED MORE THAN ONE AREA

(b) Which area, of those you have mentioned, would you most like to spend more time on?

---

26. DNA NURSING AUXILIARY, BATH NURSE/ATTENDANT, NIGHT SITTER (CODES 3,14,15 AT Q1)   X   go to 31

If you had more time, are there any particular groups of clients/patients that you would like to spend some time, or more time on?

Yes	1	ask (a)
No	2	go to 27

(a) HAND CARD C

Which groups of clients/patients?

Pregnant women	1
Mothers and new babies	2
Under 5's	3
School children	4
One parent families	5
Elderly living alone	6
Elderly (generally)	7
Mentally handicapped	8
Physically handicapped	9
Mentally ill	10
Terminally ill	11
Post-operative/Hospital discharges	12
Ethnic minorities	13
Relatives of clients/patients	14
Other (specify)	15

CODE ALL THAT APPLY

ENTER CODE FROM ABOVE

IF MENTIONED MORE THAN ONE GROUP

(b) Which group, of those you have mentioned, would you most like to spend some time, or more time, on?

28. What about clinics (screening and other types), would you like to extend this aspect of your work if you had the time?

Yes 1 ask (a)
No   2 go to 29

(a) What sorts of clinic would you do?
HAND CARD H

Antenatal,postnatal,relaxation,psychoprophylaxis	1
Well baby, infant welfare, child health	2
Developmental assessment	3
Immunisation and vaccination	4
Parentcraft/Mothercraft	5
Family planning	6
Well woman, cytology	7
Hearing and vision screening	8
School medicals	9
GP surgery sessions	10
Slimming/obesity	11
Blood pressure screening	12
Other (specify)	13

CODE ALL THAT APPLY

IF MORE THAN ONE CLINIC MENTIONED

(b) Which type of clinic, of those you have mentioned, would you most like to spend more time on?

ENTER CODE FROM ABOVE [ ]

29. If you had more time, would you like to do more studying or attend more courses related to your job?

Yes 1
No   2

30. Thinking about the way you work at the moment would you say you are a member of a primary health care team or not?

Yes 1
No   2

31. I am going to ask now about communications with staff who are involved in health care in the community. Please choose from the answers printed on this card.

HAND CARD I

On the whole, how would you assess your contacts and liaison about individual clients/patients with:-

	VERY GOOD	GOOD	FAIR	POOR	VERY POOR	DK	DNA/ NONE
						SPONTANEOUS ONLY	
a doctors involved in the care of your individual clients/patients?	1	2	3	4	5	6	7
b other primary health care staff who care for your clients/patients?	1	2	3	4	5	6	7
c other (SPECIFY TYPE OF NURSE - SEE Q1)?	1	2	3	4	5	6	7
d your supervisor?	1	2	3	4	5	6	7
e social services staff?	1	2	3	4	5	6	7

How would you assess the opportunities for more general meetings with:-

	VERY GOOD	GOOD	FAIR	POOR	VERY POOR	DK	DNA/ NONE
f other primary health care staff involved in the care of your clients/patients?	1	2	3	4	5	6	7
g nursing officers and other staff in the district?	1	2	3	4	5	6	7

32. DNA NURSING AUXILIARY, BATH NURSE/ATTENDANT,
    NIGHT SITTER   (CODES 3,14,15 AT Q1)   x   go to 33

How would you assess the following things in your current work?

Please choose from the answers printed on this card.

HAND CARD I

	VERY GOOD	GOOD	FAIR	POOR	VERY POOR	SPONTANEOUS ONLY DK	SPONTANEOUS ONLY DNA/NONE
a The opportunity to get to know your clients/patients?	1	2	3	4	5	6	7
b The opportunity to get to know GPs and their methods of working?	1	2	3	4	5	6	7
c Access to clients'/patients' records?	1	2	3	4	5	6	7
d Quality of client/patient care?	1	2	3	4	5	6	7
e Continuity of client/patient care?	1	2	3	4	5	6	7
f Your knowledge of the geographical area you work in?	1	2	3	4	5	6	7
g The opportunity to get to know clients'/patients' families?	1	2	3	4	5	6	7
h The opportunity to discuss clients/patients with doctors?	1	2	3	4	5	6	7

33. Is there anything else you would like to say about your work?

    O

CLASSIFICATION

34. What was your age last birthday?

    Under 20   1
    20 - 29   2
    30 - 39   3
    40 - 49   4
    50 - 59   5
    60 or more   6

35. Are you:-

    Married   1
    Widowed   2
    Divorced   3
    Separated   4
    or Single?   5

36. SEX   OBSERVE

    Female   1
    Male   2

THANK INFORMANT

RECORD TIME TAKEN TO COMPLETE THE INTERVIEW ....

EXPLAIN HOW TO COMPLETE THE DIARY:-

        RECORD FIRST DAY   Day
        OF DIARY RECORDING   Month

RECORD TIME TAKEN TO EXPLAIN DIARY ....

S1141 - SURVEY OF NURSES WORKING

IN THE COMMUNITY - DIARY

Please complete the diary for seven consecutive days starting

on _____   _____   _____
        DAY   DATE   MONTH

Return the completed diary in

the envelope provided

Many thanks in advance for your

help with this survey

SERIAL
NUMBER

UPPER PART OF RECORD FORM

Start each day on a new page and ring the day of the week.

For the FIRST page of each day please also complete sections (i), (ii), and (iii) as follows:

(i)   Record to the nearest half day whether you were working, on annual leave, off sick, at a course or conference or off duty.

(ii)   Record whether you were on call at any time during the period of 24 hours. If you were, then tick the hours you were on call on the a.m. and p.m. scales and below this enter the total number of hours on call.

(iii)   Record whether you were accompanied and, if so, whether this was for the whole day or only part of it.

If you continue onto a second or subsequent page please remember to ring the day of the week.

LOWER PART OF RECORD FORM

Complete one entry in the diary for each change of client/patient when out on visits, for each major change of activity when in the office or at home, or for each new clinic session if you are doing a series of clinics. (If a lot of your time is spent visiting, since most visits will probably be to one client, you will usually make an entry in the record book for each change of location). Start the diary each day at the time you begin being paid, or with the first work activity if this is earlier. Account for the WHOLE of the time for which you are officially working (whether on day or night duty) and also record any work activities in your off duty and on call time.

(iv)   In the first two columns enter the time that you started out for the location recorded and the length of time taken by your journey. If no travelling was involved then the first column should contain the time your work activity/clinic session began and the second column should be left blank. In the third column you should enter the total amount of time taken by the activities or clinic session. (This will often be the total time at that location – hence the column heading). Finally in this section record the location using a code from the list of codes above the record form.

(v) Record each of the activities you carried out, using codes from the list. Please note that the sum of the times given in section (v) should equal the time you have entered in the third column of (iv). If you should happen to carry out more than 5 activities continue on the next line leaving sections (iv), (vi) and (vii) blank on the continuation line.

We do not expect you to time each activity that you carry out but to categorize your activities and divide the total time spent in each location as accurately as possible so that the proportion of time spent on different activities is reflected.

(vi) Record client/patient details whenever you have contact with a client and for case conferences but not for clinic sessions.

All four columns of this section should be completed using codes from the list. Please note that code 01 is entered in the household type column when it is not a home visit since household details are then inapplicable.

When you discuss the health and welfare of a person or child with the person caring for him/her, the person or child being cared for should be recorded as the primary client. We leave it to your discretion as to when a visit should be recorded as having two or more primary clients and therefore have more than one entry in the diary.

(vii) Obviously this section should be left blank except when doing clinics. Enter the code from the list for the type of clinic and the number of patients/clients seen in each session.

Whenever you use an other specify code please enter details at the relevant space at the bottom of the record form.

Please do not leave blank lines in a day's record.

Please aim to fill the diary in throughout the day or at least to keep relevant notes to enable you to complete it at the end of each day.

LOCATION

01 Client's/patient's home or doorstep (include homeless family unit and sheltered housing)
02 Your own home
03 Health Centre
04 GP Premises
05 AHA premises
06 Hospital
07 Local authority home, Part III accom, private homes
08 School
09 In the street/supermarket/shops/P.O.
10 Chemist
11 Church/village hall
12 Nursery, play group, childminder
13 Club, day centre
14 Off duty location (exc. your own home)
15 Other (specify)

ACTIVITY

Non-clinical

01 No access visit, waiting, no reply
02 Clerical and administrative related to own job:
Filing, checking clerical data
Mileage claims
Kalamazoo
Work list, work plan
Write letters
Survey time
03 Clerical and administrative related to clients/patients:
Requests for equipment, aids, prescriptions, services etc
Clients'/patients' reports
Clients/patients notes
Client/patient register
04 Telephone calls
05 Meeting/consultation/liaison visits/case conference/court appearances
06 Training, teaching, supervision (given/received):
Own training - in service, Study time, course, conference, research, discussions with supervisor
Teaching/supervision - aides, auxiliaries, students and student reports
07 Preparation and collection of equipment, supplies, uniform, car etc
08 Reception duty (GP nurses)
09 Other non-clinical (specify)

Activities with patients/clients

Technical tests, assessments, screening and surveillance:
10 Scalp inspection
Vision testing
Audiometry, hearing test
Cervical smear
Taking swabs, blood/urine/faeces sample
Blood pressure
Pregnancy, skin testing
Weight, height, temperature, pulse, respiration
11 ECG
Breast palpation, examination
Ante or post-natal examination
Child development, observation
Health surveillance
Technical Procedures:
12 Injection, vaccination, immunisation
13 Eye/ear treatments, syringing
Inserting/removing stiches, plaster of paris, cervical collar
Dressings, care of pressure sores
Enema, rectal suppository, washout, manual removal
Vaginal suppository, pessary, douche
Catheterisation, bladder washout
Stoma care
Rehabilitation exercises
14 Home/GP unit delivery, attending minor ops
Other nursing care:
15 Routine nursing care, bathing, prevention of incontinence/pressure sores
16 Other personal care:
Help with lavatory, commode, bed pan
Help with washing, dressing, nappy changing
Care for hair, nails, feet
Feed or give medicine
17 Home help type care:
Prepare food and drinks
Housework, washing clothes, dishes etc
Shopping, collecting pension, benefits, prescriptions
18 Supervision of patient/client
19 Assessment visits for home conditions/social/needs for equipment etc
Delivering and instructing in use of aids/equipment
20 Other clinical (specify)

Advice, counselling, reassurance, education

21 Pregnancy, labour, family planning, vasectomy, sterilisation, abortion
22 Diet, nutrition, infant feeding, immunisation, vaccination
23 Parentcraft/children - development, management, abuse, adoption, fostering
24 Personal, emotional, social problems eg marital, bereavement, housing, financial
25 Physical health problems inc.
26 Mental health problems inc. addiction, alcoholism, depression
27 Health education - general
28 Advice to relatives - nursing care etc.
29 Reassurance - general
30 Social - chatting and listening
31 Other (specify)

CLIENT/PATIENT DETAILS

AGE AND SEX

01 Up to 1 ⎤
02 1-4   ⎥ child
03 5-15   ⎦

11 16-19
12 20-29
13 30-44
14 45-54 ⎤ woman
15 55-64 ⎥
16 65-74 ⎥
17 75-84 ⎥
18 85+   ⎦

21 16-19
22 20-29
23 30-44
24 45-54 ⎤ man
25 55-64 ⎥
26 65-74 ⎥
27 75-84 ⎥
28 85+   ⎦

31 Children
32 Young & middle aged adults
33 The elderly ⎤ Groups
34 Whole family ⎥
35 Other mixtures (specify) ⎦

HOUSEHOLD TYPE

01 Does not apply - not home visit
02 Lone adult - with or without children
03 Adults only - all aged 65+
04 All other household types
05 Don't know

TYPE OF CLIENT/PATIENT

01 Expectant mother
02 Maternity - within 28 days of delivery
03 Baby, toddler or child and person caring for it
04 School child and/or person caring for it
05 Post-operative, hospital discharge (last 28 days)
06 Terminal/deteriorating
07 Physical handicap also inc. arthritis, rheumatism, paralysis other limitations on mobility etc.
08 Mental handicap, subnormality
09 Mental illness inc. depression, senile dementia, confusion personality disorder etc
10 Chest disease inc. TB, bronchitis, pneumonia and infections etc.
11 Cardio-vascular disease inc. heart, stroke and hypertension patients
12 Skin inc. ulcers, pressure sores, etc
13 Diabetic
14 Elderly - general frailty or no specific condition or condition not known
15 Other medical/surgical (specify)
16 Group visit eg. old people's home, community groups inc wardens
17 Problem family
18 Other (specify)

WHO INITIATED THIS CONTACT

01 Primary visit to new born baby
02 Yourself - first visit
03 Yourself - routine, follow-up
04 Client/patient or their family
05 GP
06 Other member of practice team
07 Other community nursing staff
08 Hospital
09 School health service/teacher
10 Social services staff
11 Voluntary agency/worker
12 No-one ie chance meeting
13 Other (specify)

TYPE OF CLINIC SESSION

01 Ante natal and post-natal inc relaxation, psychoprophylaxis and booking clinic
02 Well baby, infant welfare, child health
03 Developmental assessment
04 Immunisation and vaccination
05 Rubella vaccination
06 Mothercraft/parentcraft
07 Family planning
08 Well woman, cytology
09 Hearing and vision
10 School medicals/hygiene inspection
11 Health education sessions
12 GP surgery sessions
13 Other (specify)

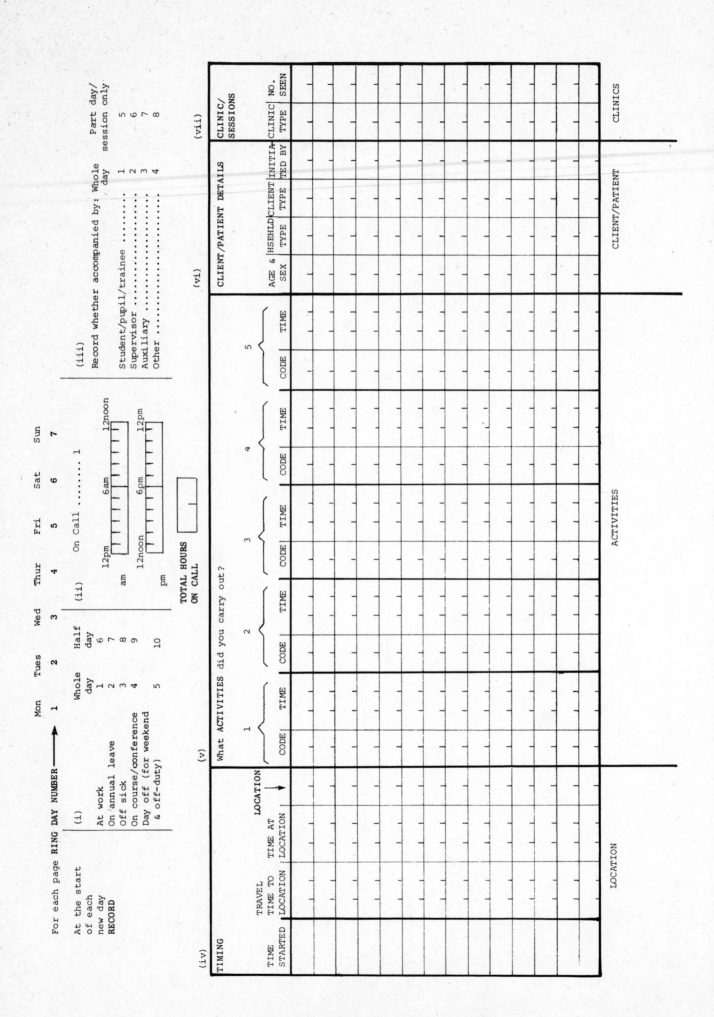

For each page RING DAY NUMBER ⟶

	Mon	Tues	Wed	Thur	Fri	Sat	Sun
	1	2	3	4	5	6	7

At the start of each new day RECORD

(i)

	Whole day	Half day		Part day/ session only
At work	1	6		
On annual leave	2	7		
Off sick	3	8		
On course/conference	4	9		
Day off (for weekend & off-duty)	5	10		

(iii) Record whether accompanied by:

	Whole day	Part day/ session only
Student/pupil/trainee	1	5
Supervisor	2	6
Auxiliary	3	7
Other	4	8

(ii)

am   12pm   6am   12noon

pm   12noon   6pm   12pm

On Call 1

TOTAL HOURS ON CALL

(iv) TIMING

TIME STARTED | TRAVEL TIME TO LOCATION | TIME AT LOCATION | LOCATION ⟶

LOCATION

(v) What ACTIVITIES did you carry out?

1		2		3		4		5	
CODE	TIME	CODE	TIME	CODE	TIME	CODE	TIME	CODE	TIME

ACTIVITIES

(vi) CLIENT/PATIENT DETAILS

AGE & SEX	HSEHLD TYPE	CLIENT TYPE	INITIA-TED BY

CLIENT/PATIENT

(vii) CLINIC/ SESSIONS

CLINIC TYPE	NO. SEEN

CLINICS

Printed in England for Her Majesty's Stationery Office
by Robendene Ltd, Amersham, Bucks.
Dd 717530 C 13 4/82